SOLO's Field Guide to Wilderness First Aid

Wilderness, Marine, Rural, Disaster, International

"Beyond the Golden Hour"

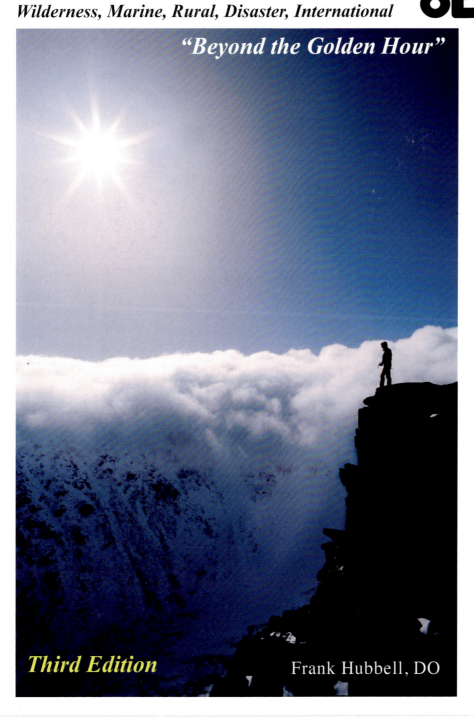

Third Edition

Frank Hubbell, DO

SOLO'S FIELD GUIDE TO WILDERNESS FIRST AID
Third Edition

Published by:
TMC Books/Stonehearth Open Learning Opportunities
731 Tasker Hill Rd., Conway, NH 03818
info@TMCBooks.com
http://www.TMCbooks.com
http://www.soloschools.com
082907

All rights reserved. No part of this book may be reproduced or transmitted in any form or by any means, electronic or mechanical, including photocopying, recording, or by any information storage or retrieval system without written permission from the publisher, except for the inclusion of brief quotations in a review.

© Copyright 2005, 2006, May 2007, August 2007, Third Edition—May 2014
by Franklin R. Hubbell, DO

ISBN: 978-0-9826539-7-5

Printed in Canada
Friesens Corporation, Altona, Manitoba

This book is dedicated

to my co-founder, co-director, and wife, Lee Frizzell.

For without her heart, patience, and kind spirit, none of this would exist.

And to all the Good Samaritans who have the heart to stop and help.

Jesus replied and said, "A certain man was going down from Jerusalem to Jericho; and he fell among robbers, and they stripped him and beat him, and went off leaving him half dead.

"And by chance a certain priest was going down on that road, and when he saw him, he passed by on the other side.

"And likewise a Levite also, when he came to the place and saw him, passed by on the other side.

"But a certain Samaritan, who was on a journey, came upon him; and when he saw him, he felt compassion, and came to him, and bandaged up his wounds, pouring oil and wine on them; and he put him on his own beast, and brought him to an inn, and took care of him."

Luke 10:30-34
NAS

SOLO's Field Guide to Wilderness First Aid

The SOLO Field Guide to Wilderness First Aid is the manual that accompanies SOLO's two-day course of the same name. The Wilderness First Aid (WFA) course was created out of the direct experience of the founders of SOLO and is designed by and for the "outdoor enthusiast:" whether hiker, climber, skier, kayaker, canoeist, or sailor. It is for the adventurous who may find themselves away from immediate help and may have to rely on their own skills to survive and thrive if an emergency should arise.

First offered in 1974 under the name of the Mountain Rescue Seminar, the course next became Backcountry Medicine, and eventually Wilderness First Aid. The course has continued to evolve over the past 40 years, through over a thousand programs, and more than 300,000 students.

A jam-packed, fast-paced course, WFA covers a variety of topics including how to recognize and manage common medical problems along with rare but life-threatening emergencies, environmental emergencies, and most importantly, prevention of these problems. This textbook is intended to be a true field guide that our students can carry with them throughout their training with SOLO and use as a reference later.

This course is recognized by the American Camping Association as the minimal standard for camp counselors, both day hiking and overnight hiking leaders. For professional outdoor leaders doing multi-day trips or expedition-level mountaineering, this course is a good start and will help prepare students for SOLO's Wilderness First Responder or Wilderness Emergency Medical Technician certification programs.

Table of Contents

INTRODUCTION:
   What is a WFA? *The "wilderness" in wilderness first aid* -------- 6

CHAPTER ONE: RESPONSE AND ASSESSMENT
   Universal Precautions: *Body Substance Isolation* -------- 10
   Anatomy of a Crisis: *The Patient Assessment System* -------- 12
   Patient Assessment Checklist -------- 28
   Patient Lifting and Moving Techniques: *How to move a wounded friend* -------- 31
   Shock -------- 34

CHAPTER TWO: ORTHOPEDICS: TRAUMA—MUSCULOSKELETAL INJURIES
   Anatomy of the Musculoskeletal System: *How is it organized and how does it work?* -------- 38
   Sprain and Strains: *How to recognize and treat the most common injuries* -------- 40
   Principles of Fracture Care: *How to recognize and treat a fracture* -------- 41
   Spinal Cord Injury Management: *How to clear the spine; if you can't, how to treat* -------- 44

CHAPTER THREE: ENVIRONMENTAL EMERGENCIES & SURVIVAL SKILLS
   The Human Animal: *The physical limitations of the human animal* -------- 48
   Cold-Related Injuries: *Hypothermia and Frostbite* -------- 52
   Heat-Related Injuries: *Dehydration, Heat Exhaustion, and Heat Stroke* -------- 58
   North American Bites and Stings: *Bugs and snakes* -------- 60
   Lightning -------- 62
   Backcountry Essentials: Bivouac, & Survival Skills: *How to stay put and get help* -------- 64

CHAPTER FOUR: SOFT TISSUE INJURIES & MEDICAL EMERGENCIES
   Trauma—Soft Tissue Injuries:
      Soft Tissue Injuries and Wound Management: *How to manage common injuries* -------- 70
      Bandaging Skills: *How to make a bandage to support a wound dressing* -------- 80
   Medical Emergencies & Critical Care: *Rare but potentially life-threatening problems*
      Change in Level of Consciousness: brain, oxygen, sugar, temperature, pressure, seizures -------- 82
      Shortness of Breath: breathing, pneumothorax, asthma, severe allergic reaction -------- 83
      Asthma -------- 84
      Chest Pain: pulse, heart attack -------- 84
      Anaphylaxis -------- 85

APPENDICES:
   What is SOLO? *Stonehearth Open Learning Opportunities* -------- 87
   Chapter Quizzes -------- 89
   Blank SOAPnotes -------- 93
   Certificate of Completion -------- 97

Editor's Note: *We extend our apologies to grammarians for the often unorthodox use of punctuation marks and capital letters and for the intentional lack of agreement between pronouns and their antecedents.*

THE "WILDERNESS" IN WILDERNESS FIRST AID:

WHAT IS "WILDERNESS" AND WHY IS IT SO CHALLENGING TO THE EMERGENCY CAREGIVER?

In the world of pre-hospital medicine, the term "wilderness" or "extended care" is defined as any time a patient is more than an hour from definitive (hospital ER) care. The critical first hour after an injury occurs is called the "Golden Hour."

In the wilderness setting it is very easy to consume an hour in a rescue effort. When someone becomes sick or injured a chain of events has to occur to get the patient out of the woods and into the hospital, and it is more than simply calling 911. Commonly, someone has to hike out and notify EMS; then EMS has to respond to the trailhead, hike back in to the patient, treat and package the patient, carry them out to the waiting ambulance, and finally transport them to the hospital. A general rule of thumb to estimate the total rescue time from injury to the hospital is one hour of effort for every quarter-mile from the road.

Distance and Time: it's farther and longer than you think.

- Rapid notification for help is usually impossible.
- Someone may have to go for help on foot. What information should they carry out?
- The response by the rescue team is prolonged; they usually have to walk in. What will you do until they arrive?
- Provision of emergency care is clearly outside the "Golden Hour."

The Environment: can easily turn hostile.

- Cold, wet, snow, or darkness can delay rescuers even longer.
- Poor weather conditions can be a direct threat to the safety of rescuers, the patient, and others with the patient.
- Poor weather conditions may eliminate the possibility of access by helicopter.
- It can be much more difficult to take care of yourself, the patient, and anyone else on the scene.

INTRODUCTION

Think about the Terrain: travel can be hazardous and slow.
- Access to the patient might require special skills such as rock climbing ability or experience.
- Terrain features such as deep snow, deep mud, or even a steep trail can further slow rescuers.
- Terrain features may even present extreme dangers in the form of avalanches or flooded river crossings.
- There may be route-finding difficulties.

Equipment and Resources: maximize efficiency to minimize weight.
- Is the group to be rescued prepared for the conditions?
- Is the responding team "wilderness" trained and prepared for the conditions?
- The group must know how to improvise equipment.
- Limited equipment and access to resources is the norm.

Specialized Training and Wilderness Knowledge: get smart.
- Map and compass and route-finding skills, search and rescue skills.
- Weather forecasting skills.
- Bivouac skills.
- Technical rescue skills, ropes and knots, water rescue skills.
- Understanding long-term patient care.
- Helicopter rescue training.

For all of these reasons wilderness care providers are expected to follow and to perform at a different standard of care than a care provider in an urban setting. As implied, someone learning wilderness first aid may need to learn and master a number of skills that are not directly related to patient care. They may also be expected to manage an injury differently than a caregiver in an urban environment simply because the wilderness care provider may be staying with the patient for a long time while waiting for help to arrive, and possibly while the patient is being transported to definitive care.

NOTES

CHAPTER ONE

RESPONSE AND ASSESSMENT
What happened?

BODY SUBSTANCE ISOLATION (BSI):
Also referred to as Total Fluid Precautions or Universal Precautions

In providing emergency medical care you can be exposed to infectious disease agents, and you need to know how to protect yourself against these disease-causing organisms.

Modes of Transmission

DIRECT CONTACT
The spread of disease by direct contact with the blood or other body substances of an infected individual (saliva, sputum, blood, urine, feces, secretions).

INDIRECT CONTACT
The spread of disease from one individual to another by touching a contaminated inanimate object (door knob, clothing, stretcher, countertop, etc.) and then transferring the pathogen to mouth or eyes with the now contaminated hands.

AIRBORNE
The spread of disease by infected droplets of saliva or sputum expelled into the air by coughing or sneezing and then being inhaled by another person.

VECTOR
The spread of disease by blood-sucking insects, such as mosquitoes, fleas, or ticks.

WATERBORNE
The spread of disease by the consumption of contaminated water, usually contaminated with human waste, the "oral fecal route."

RESPONSE AND ASSESSMENT

Our primary defense is behavior: we take precautions to prevent contamination. PREVENTION equals BEHAVIOR.

GLOVES OR WATERPROOF BARRIER

To prevent DIRECT CONTACT, establish a barrier before any potential exposure to body fluids.

HAND-WASHING

To prevent patient-to-patient and hand-to-mouth transfer of pathogens by INDIRECT CONTACT, wash hands before and after any patient contact.

MASKS

To prevent AIRBORNE spread, put on a surgical mask before any potential exposure to airborne pathogens, especially tuberculosis (put a mask on the patient, too, if possible).

INSECT REPELLENT, MOSQUITO NETTING, CLOTHING

To prevent the transmission of disease by blood-sucking insects, use insect repellents (Permethrin), wear protective clothing, sleep under mosquito netting, and do tick checks.

WATER PURIFICATION

To prevent waterborne illnesses always make and drink potable water by boiling, use of water filters, chemicals (iodine or chlorine), or the use of UVC light (Steripen).

11

THE ANATOMY OF A CRISIS: THE PATIENT ASSESSMENT SYSTEM

What would you do if you were hiking along and were the first one to arrive at the scene of an accident?
- How would you find out what is wrong and what has happened?
- How do you tell how badly hurt the injured person is?
- Do you go for help?
- Do you try to help the injured person?
- What should you do?

The method used is STOP and Survey referred to as *The Patient Assessment System* which consists of a list of questions and tasks that need to be performed in order to ascertain what happened and what you are going to do about it.
- These questions and tasks are arranged by priority and should be done in order.
- You should not move on to the next task until the one you are on has been successfully completed.

Part 1—STOP—SCENE SURVEY: Is the scene safe?
- Are you safe?
- Is everyone else safe?
- Is the patient safe?
- What happened? (Mechanism of Injury—MOI)
- How do you safely approach the victim?
- What is your general impression of the situation's seriousness?

Part 2—STOP—PRIMARY SURVEY: Are they alive?

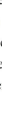

- Approach and Assess—Are they conscious and can they speak?
- Airway—Do they have an open airway?
- Breathing—Are they breathing?
- Breathing—How well are they breathing?
- Circulation—Do they have a pulse?
- Circulation—Are they bleeding?
- D: Deformity—Are there any obvious deformities?
- D: Disability—Is their neck or back at risk of injury?
- E: Environment—Can they stay where they are?
- E: Everyone Else—Is everyone else high and dry and safe?

RESPONSE AND ASSESSMENT

Part 3—STOP—SECONDARY SURVEY: How Are They?

- What happened?—the History of Present Illness
- How well are they doing?—Vital Signs
- What are their injuries?—Patient Exam
- What is their past medical history?—AMPLE History
- What is your patient care plan? —SOAPnote

Part 4—STOP—RESCUE SURVEY: Do you need help?

- What is your plan to get help?
- Who is being sent for help?
- What do you need to do to protect the patient while waiting for help to arrive?
- What do you need to do to protect yourselves while waiting for help to arrive?
- Is the scene safe for the group?
- Perform on-going assessment; re-SOAP every 15 minutes.

13

WILDERNESS FIRST AID

PATIENT ASSESSMENT SYSTEM
in detail

To survey something is to examine it closely and ascertain its condition. In this system of STOP and Survey, the intent is to take the time to STOP and take a deep breath before closely examining and ascertaining the patient's condition. A survey is organized in a logical step-by-step process that allows you to gather the information and respond in an orderly manner.

PART 1: STOP—SCENE SURVEY: Is the Scene Safe?

- Are you OK, and are you going to stay OK?
- Are the others OK, and are they going to stay OK?
- Is the victim of this crisis OK, and are they going to stay OK?
- What happened? What was the mechanism of injury (MOI)?
- How do you safely approach the victim?
- What is your general impression of how serious this is?

To accomplish all this Scene Survey:

 Stop. Stand still, take a deep breath, and ask yourself, "Am I OK?" If not, do something about it! **Go.**

 Stop. Tell everyone else to STOP, stand still, take a deep breath and ask themselves, "Am I OK?" If not, do something about it! Don't allow anyone to run off to check the victim or to get help. **Go.**

 Stop. Is the victim OK? First speak or call out to them, even if you cannot see them or get to them. Ask them if they are all right. Hopefully, they will answer; even if they say that they are not all right, at least you know they are alive, have an open airway, are breathing, and have a pulse. **Go.**

 Stop. Ask yourself, "What happened?" "What was the mechanism of injury?" **Go.**

 Stop. Survey the victim's situation. While figuring out how to safely get to them, keep talking to them. Be positive, keep encouraging them, tell them to lie still, that help is on the way. **Go.**

 Stop. As you approach the victim, survey their position. Ask yourself, "Can they stay where they are, or are they in imminent danger and need to be moved?" **Go.**

 Stop. What is your impression of the victim? As you approach the victim (they do not become your patient until you lay your hands on them), develop a general impression of how serious the situation seems to be, based on the position they are lying in, how they look, whether they are conscious, bleeding, etc. **Go.**

RESPONSE AND ASSESSMENT

PART 2: STOP—PRIMARY SURVEY:
Are they alive, and are they going to stay alive?

Approach and Assess—Are they conscious and can they speak?
Airway—Do they have an open airway?

Breathing—Are they breathing?
Breathing—How well are they breathing?

Circulation—Do they have a pulse?
Circulation—Are they bleeding?

Deformity—Are there any obvious deformities?
Disability—Is their neck or back at risk of injury?

Environment—Can they stay where they are?
Everyone Else—How is everyone else in the group doing?

The primary survey is a rapid assessment of all the vital functions necessary to support life: the central nervous system, the respiratory system, and the circulatory system.

- It also takes into consideration how the environment is impacting on the patient.
- If there is a problem, you do not move on to the next step until that problem is solved.
- Each aspect of the primary survey is explored by looking, listening, and feeling.

Look, Listen, & Feel—the keys to the primary survey

15

Approach and Assess—Are they conscious, and can they speak?

Look—Are they awake; are their eyes open; what position are they lying in?

Listen—Speak to them. Do they speak back?

Feel—What is your general impression of the situation?

- Upon arrival, kneel down next to the patient's head and place a hand on their forehead to hold their head still.
- This not only protects the cervical spine, it also makes physical contact with them, providing "the human touch."
- Continue to speak to them even if they are unconscious.
- The first question you ask is are they conscious or unconscious? If they are conscious, can they speak?
- If they are conscious, ask them to lie still until you have had a chance to check them out.
- Ask the obvious questions: "Are you all right?" "Where does is hurt?" "Do you know what happened?"
- If they are unconscious, you need to make sure that they have an open airway.
- To test for LOC, apply a painful, but harmless, stimulus.

Airway—Do they have an open airway?

Look—Is there anything in their airway?

Listen—Can you hear air moving in and out of the airway?

Feel—Can you feel air moving in and out of the airway?

- Lean over your unconscious patient and place your ear in front of their mouth so that you can feel and hear air moving in and out of their airway.
- If they are not breathing, inspect the airway. The most common cause of an obstructed airway is the tongue and position of the head.
- To open the airway, move the head into proper anatomical position. Tilt it slightly back (extension), and gently pull the lower jaw (mandible) forward. This moves the musculature of the tongue forward and opens the airway.
- Again, place you ear over their mouth to make sure that they are breathing.

RESPONSE AND ASSESSMENT

Breathing—Are they breathing?

Look—Is their chest wall moving as they breathe?
Listen—Can you hear breath sounds?
Feel—Can you feel air moving in and out of their mouth?

- While leaning over, with your ear in front of their mouth, listen to them breathe and make sure air is moving in and out of the airway. Listen to their breath sounds.
- If they are not breathing, give them two full breaths and check to see if they have a pulse. If they have a pulse, continue to give them one full breath every 4–5 seconds until they are breathing on their own.
- If they do not have a pulse, initiate CPR.

Breathing—How well are they breathing?

Look—What is their skin color (are they pale, ashen, blue)?
Listen—Can you hear any adventitious breath sounds such as wheezing, gurgling, or snoring, indicating a partially occluded airway, ?
Feel—Is the chest wall moving appropriately with respirations?

- If they are breathing, listen to see if they are making any adventitious breath sounds such as wheezing, snoring, gurgling, or coughing.
- If any of these sounds are heard, log roll the patient into the recovery position to help clear and maintain an open airway.
- In the recovery position gravity will drain any fluids from the airway and allow the tongue to fall forward opening the airway.
- Never tolerate any adventitious breath sounds as they indicate that the airway is at least partially occluded and the patient is not getting enough oxygen.
- Breathing includes not only whether they are breathing (is air moving in and out of the lungs), but also how well they are breathing.
- Are they breathing often enough and deeply enough to get an adequate supply of oxygen into the lungs and, therefore, into the blood.
- A normal respiratory rate is between 10–30 breaths per minute depending upon age and activity level.
- If they are not taking at least one breath every 6 seconds, 10 breaths per minute, then you need to assist ventilate with at least one full breath every 4–5 seconds.
- If their respiratory rate is greater than 1 breath every 2 seconds or 30 breaths per minute, they are breathing too fast and too shallowly to allow for good air exchange.
- Again assist ventilate them at a rate of one full breath every 4–5 seconds to improve the air exchange in the lungs.
- Now that you know they have an open airway and adequate breathing, check their pulse.

Circulation—Do they have a pulse?

Look—Is their skin pale? Are they cyanotic (bluish)?
Listen—Can you hear a heartbeat?
Feel—Can you feel a carotid pulse?

- Once you have established that they have an open airway and they are breathing, check a carotid pulse.
- This is accomplished by placing your 2nd and 3rd fingers over the center of the trachea and drawing your hand towards yourself and into the groove between the trachea and the sternocleidomastoid muscles of the neck. As you gently compress this groove, you will be able to palpate the carotid artery pulse.
- If they do not have a pulse, initiate CPR. If for some reason you cannot access or feel the carotid pulse, you can place your ear over the left side of the chest to listen for a heartbeat.

Circulation—Are they bleeding?

Look—Is there any active bleeding?
Listen—Can you hear a heartbeat?
Feel—Can you feel a carotid pulse?

- Along with determining if there is a pulse, you also need to scan the length of their body and look for any signs of obvious bleeding.
- If there are areas of blood in their clothing or blood pooling on the ground, inspect the area for any source of the bleeding.
- A minor scrape that is oozing blood can be ignored for now.
- Your concern is major bleeding from blood that is spurting from the body or rapidly flowing from a wound. This type of bleeding must be controlled.
- Apply direct pressure to the wound. Remember Body Substance Isolation (BSI) and either put on gloves or create a barrier between you and the body fluid.

Perform a "chunk check" to check for bleeding.

RESPONSE AND ASSESSMENT

Deformity—Do they have any obvious injuries or deformities?

Look—Do you see any obvious injuries or deformities?
Listen—Where are they complaining of pain?
Feel—Where does it hurt? As you touch them, where can you cause pain?

- This is referred to as a "chunk check."
- Scan the length of the body looking for any obvious deformities like angulated fractures. See if there is anything sticking out of the body that belongs inside or anything sticking into the body that belongs outside.
- Then perform a chunk check by quickly palpating the major parts of the body.
- You want to gently compress the head, the neck, the chest, the abdomen, the pelvis, and the upper legs, feeling for injuries or pain response.
- If you find any injuries, take the time to inspect the area to see if there is something that you need to deal with immediately.

Is their neck or back at risk of injury?

Look—What was the mechanism of injury (MOI)? Can they move their extremities?
Listen—Are they complaining of any neck or back pain?
Feel—Do they have normal sensation in their extremities?

- Upon arrival at the patient's side, you place a hand on the forehead to hold their head still, or you ask someone else to stabilize the cervical spine while you continue the PAS.
- If they are unconscious, or if the mechanism of injury (MOI) indicates possible injury to the spine, continue to immobilize their neck and back.
- Later after completion of the PAS, you will come back and re-examine the spine to see if you can clear it or if you need to continue immobilization of the spine.

Environment—Can they stay where they are?

Look—Where are they lying?
Listen—Are they complaining about being hot, cold, or wet?
Feel—Is their skin warm, dry, cold, or wet?

- Right from the moment you arrive at the patient's side, you have to be asking yourself if they can stay where they are or if they need to be moved.
- Whenever possible, you try to keep them lying still until you can complete the PAS and you have a good idea what the injuries are.
- However, this is not always possible, and you may have to move them without knowing the extent of the injuries.
- If a move is necessary, you have to figure out where they can be safely relocated.
- At a minimum and as soon as possible, get them onto an ensolite pad or other soft, insulating material to protect them from the ground.
- If necessary, surround them with warm insulation or provide shade.
- Eventually they will have to be moved into a shelter to protect them from the weather.

Everyone Else—How is everyone else in the group doing?

Look—How does the rest of the group look?
Listen—Is anyone complaining of being cold, wet, hungry, or thirsty?
Feel—What is the emotional status of the group?

- STOP and consider the whole group.
- How is everyone else doing?
- Is everyone warm and dry and protected from the environment?
- Keep everyone busy.

RESPONSE AND ASSESSMENT

PART 3: STOP—SECONDARY SURVEY—History of Present Illness, Vital Signs, Patient Exam, AMPLE History, SOAPnote

- What happened?—History of Present Illness
- How well are they?—Vital Signs
- What are their injuries?—Patient Exam
- What is their past medical history?—AMPLE History
- What is our patient care plan?—SOAPnote

Upon completion of the Scene Survey and the Primary Survey, the life-threatening problems have been eliminated or managed. Now you have the luxury of time to move on to the Secondary Survey and answer the question, "How hurt are they?" By taking a set of vital signs, performing a patient exam, and taking an AMPLE history, you will be able to determine the extent and severity of the injuries or illness.

History of Present Illness:
- Onset of injury or illness
- Location of pain or injury
- Quality of pain
- Quantity of pain (0 = no pain; 10 = worst pain ever)

Vital Signs

A person's ability to acquire and utilize oxygen (O_2) is the most important thing. The first responsibility is to make sure the person has an open airway, is breathing, has a pulse, and is not bleeding. Once that is established, you measure and monitor the VITAL SIGNS of the body's major systems in order to determine if a person is getting better, staying the same, or getting worse as a result of injuries, illness, or care provided.

A person can live:
- Weeks without food.
- Days without water.
- Hours in a harsh environment without shelter.
- But only SIX MINUTES without oxygen.

What vital signs tell you:
- How well your patient is doing in response to the injury.
- And how serious the injury is.

What vital signs don't tell you:
- What the specific injury is.

Vital signs set the pace:
- Take a set of vital signs every 5–15 minutes.
- They give you a picture over time of how well your patient is doing.
- They give you confidence that you are doing your job and your patient is doing well.

Vital Signs: By System

Respiratory System (airway and lungs)
The oxygen exchange system: "In with the good air and out with the bad."

- Respiratory Rate: Count the number of breaths per minute—normal: 10-30/minute
- Respiratory Effort: Observe; watch them breathe—normal: no effort
- How hard are they working to breathe?
- Ask them if they feel short of breath, or if they are having a hard time breathing.

Circulatory System (heart, blood vessels, and blood)
Transports the oxygen to every cell in the body: "Do not be still, my beating heart."

- Heart Rate: Find the pulse at the wrist and count it for a minute—normal: 50-100 beats/minute
- Effort: May use a blood pressure (bp) cuff or simply check for pulses—normal: all pulses intact
    - If you get a pulse at the wrist, there is a minimum BP of 90mmHg, enough to perfuse the entire body.
    - If you get a pulse at the femoral artery, there is a minimum BP of 70mmHg, enough to perfuse the vital organs and brain.
    - If you get a pulse at the carotid artery, there is a minimum BP of 60mmHg, enough to perfuse only the brain.

Central Nervous System (brain and spinal cord)
Uses oxygen to survive and thrive and establishes the Level of Consciousness (LOC).

- Monitor LOC with the AVPU scale—normal: awake, alert, oriented x 3

Awake: conscious: how alert are they? —"The lights are on, but is anyone home?"
- Alert and Oriented times one (x1): **person**—they only know who they are (A&O x 1 = bad).
- Alert and Oriented x 2: **place**—they know who they are and where they are (A&O x 2 = better).
- Alert and Oriented x 3: **time**—they know who they are, where they are, the day, week, & year (A&O x 3 = best).

Verbal: unconscious: but do they respond to sound?— "Hello, anyone in there?"
- Speak to them; do they react to hearing their name (attempting to speak, making movement)?
- Do they follow simple commands (blinking, moving a limb)?

Painful: unconscious: but do they respond to pain?—"That's got to hurt."
- Does a knuckle rubbed on their sternum elicit a response (guarding, groaning)?
- Is it an appropriate response to pain?

Unresponsive: unconscious, comatose.
- "No one's home."
- No response to verbal or painful stimuli.

RESPONSE AND ASSESSMENT

Integumentary System (skin):
The largest organ in the human body, responsible for thermoregulation. If there is limited oxygen, the brain will prioritize and vasoconstrict the peripheral circulation in the skin, shunting the blood away from the skin to vital organs.

Skin color: varies by individual and race.
- Is there perfusion of blood to the skin?
- Check capillary refill.
- Look at the nonpigmented areas of the body: the nail beds, under the eyelids, in the mouth.

Skin temperature and moisture: not too hot, not too cold.
- Touch their skin on the abdomen and in the axilla.
- Are they hot or cold to the touch? Are they dry, wet, or sweaty?

HEALTHY SET OF VITAL SIGNS

Vital Sign	Time (0:00)	Time (0:15)	Time (0:30)	Time (0:45)
RR & Effort	16—no effort	12—no effort	12—no effort	12—no effort
HR & Effort (BP by palp)	80 + radial pulse	72 + radial pulse	60 + radial pulse	60 + radial pulse
LOC	A&O x 3	A&O x 3	A&O x 3	A&O x 3
Skin	warm & moist	warm & moist	warm & moist	warm & moist

VITAL SIGNS IN SHOCK

Vital Sign	Time (0:00)	Time (0:15)	Time (0:30)	Time (0:45)
RR & Effort	16—no effort	12—no effort	20—no effort	30—with effort
HR & Effort (BP by palp)	80 + radial pulse	72 + radial pulse	80 + radial pulse	100 + carotid pulse
LOC	A&O x 3	A&O x 3	A&O x 3 + anxious	A&O x 2 + anxious
Skin	warm & moist	warm & moist	pale & cool	pale, cool, & clammy

Patient Exam—The principles of a thorough search for trouble

- Hands-on, head-to-toe exam that locates the injuries.
- Done in much the same way as a good massage.
- One person does the entire exam.
- Start at the head; then do: neck—chest—abdomen—legs—arms—back.
- Talk with the patient; explain what you are doing.
- If they complain of pain, ask where it hurts.
- Avoid unnecessary movement.
- History of Present Illness—get a thorough history of what happened.

Principles of the Patient Exam—you are trying to discover all possible injuries by:

INSPECTION: Look for bleeding & wounds, impaled objects, deformities.

CIRCULATION: Check all four extremities for pulses.

C

COMPARISON: Check symmetry of body parts.

SENSATION: Check all four extremities for sensation.

S

PALPATION: Is there tenderness in muscles, bones, or joints?

MOTION: Check all four extremities for the ability to move.

M

24

RESPONSE AND ASSESSMENT

HEAD: Inspect scalp, face, eyes, nose, mouth, ears.

NECK: Palpate cervical spine, inspect trachea.

CHEST: Palpate clavicles, shoulder, and compress the rib cage.

ABDOMEN: Compress the abdomen in the center.

PELVIS: Compress the pelvis front to back and laterally.

LEGS: Palpate the muscles and ask patient to flex the joints.

ARMS: Palpate the muscles and ask patient to flex their joints.

BACK: Palpate the length of the back.

25

AMPLE History

Everyone has a past medical history that others may not be aware of. This medical history can be very important and can be a factor in providing proper medical care. Use the simple mnemonic of AMPLE to remind yourself of the appropriate questions to ask your patients about their medical history.

Allergies
- To medications, foods, insects, etc.
- What happens and how is it treated?

Medications
- What medications are they taking (both prescription and over-the-counter)?
- Have they taken their meds today? How often and how much?

Previous Injury or Illness
- Any recent or past injury or illness that could contribute to the current problem?

Last Input and Output
- When was the last time they ate or drank?
- What did they eat and drink?
- When was the last time they voided or had a bowel movement?

Events leading up to the crisis
- What led up to or occurred just prior to the critical event?

Allergies?

Medications?

History?

Last in, last out

What happened??

RESPONSE AND ASSESSMENT

SOAPnote

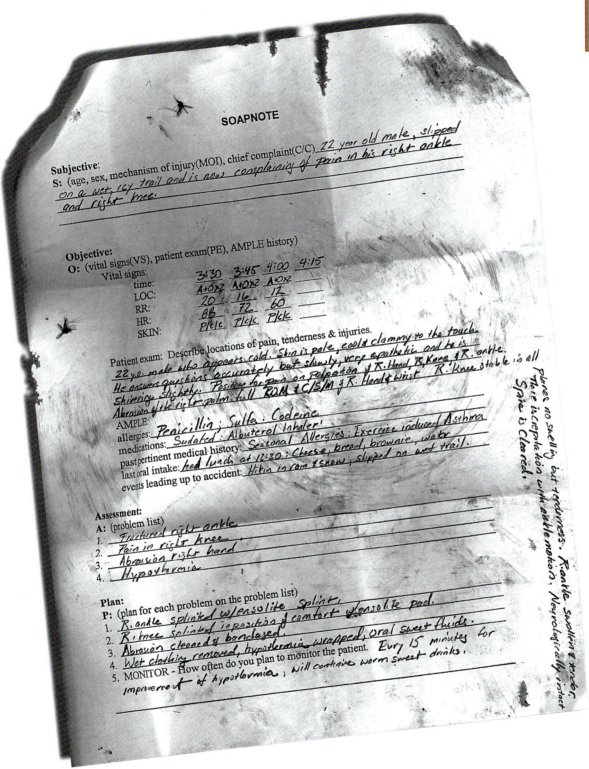

SOAPNOTE

Subjective:
S: (age, sex, mechanism of injury(MOI), chief complaint(C/C): 22 year old male, slipped on a wet, icy trail and is now complaining of pain in his right ankle and right knee.

Objective:
O: (vital signs(VS), patient exam(PE), AMPLE history)

Vital signs:				
time:	3:30	3:45	4:00	4:15
LOC:	A+Ox2	A+Ox2	A+Ox2	
RR:	20	16	12	
HR:	88	72	60	
SKIN:	P|c|c	P|c|c	P|c|c	

Patient exam: Describe locations of pain, tenderness & injuries.
22 y.o. male who appears cold. Skin is pale, cool & clammy to the touch. He answers questions accurately but slowly, very apathetic and he is shivering slightly. Positive for pain on palpation of R.Hand, R.Knee & R. ankle. Abrasion L is r-palm. full ROM & C/S/M of R. Hand & Wrist. R. knee stable is all

AMPLE:
allergies: Penicillin, Sulfa, Codeine
medications: Sudafed, Albuterol Inhaler.
past pertinent medical history: Seasonal Allergies; Exercise induced Asthma
last oral intake: had lunch at 12:30. Cheese, bread, brownie, water
events leading up to accident: Hikin in rain & snow, slipped on wet trail.

[margin note: Planes no swelling but + tenderness. R.ankle swollen & tender. There is crepitation with ankle motion. Neurologically intact Spine is Cleared.]

Assessment:
A: (problem list)
1. Fractured right ankle
2. Pain in right knee
3. Abrasion right hand
4. Hypothermia

Plan:
P: (plan for each problem on the problem list)
1. R.ankle splinted w/ensolite splint.
2. R.knee splinted in position of comfort w/ensolite pad.
3. Abrasion cleaned & bandaged.
4. Wet clothing removed, hypothermia wrapped, oral sweet fluids.
5. MONITOR - How often do you plan to monitor the patient. Every 15 minutes for improvement of hypothermia, will continue warm sweet drinks.

PATIENT ASSESSMENT CHECK LIST

SCENE SIZE-UP:

- [ ] Is the SCENE SAFE?
- [ ] Is the PATIENT SAFE?
- [ ] BSI?

PRIMARY SURVEY:

- [ ] Is the patient CONSCIOUS?
- [ ] Do they have an OPEN AIRWAY?
- [ ] Are they BREATHING?
- [ ] Are they BLEEDING?
- [ ] Do they have a PULSE?
- [ ] Are there any serious injuries on the CHUNK CHECK?
- [ ] Do they need to be MOVED?
- [ ] Do they need to be DE-CRUMPLED?
- [ ] Do you need to protect them from the ENVIRONMENT?

SECONDARY SURVEY—VITAL SIGNS:

- [ ] What is their RESPIRATORY RATE & EFFORT?
- [ ] What is their HEART RATE & EFFORT?
- [ ] What is their LEVEL OF CONSCIOUSNESS?
- [ ] What is their SKIN COLOR, TEMPERATURE, & MOISTURE?

RESPONSE AND ASSESSMENT

SECONDARY SURVEY—PATIENT EXAM:

- [ ] HEAD—scalp, face, eyes, nose, mouth
- [ ] NECK—spine, trachea
- [ ] CHEST—clavicles, shoulders, ribs
- [ ] ABDOMEN—compress the abdomen
- [ ] PELVIS—compress the pelvis, anterior/posterior and lateral
- [ ] LEGS—circulation, sensation, and motion
- [ ] ARMS—circulation, sensation, and motion
- [ ] BACK—log roll and palpate the length of the spine

SECONDARY SURVEY—AMPLE HISTORY:

- [ ] ALLERGY—allergy to drugs, foods, insects, etc.
- [ ] MEDS—prescription and non-prescription drugs
- [ ] PREVIOUS—significant past medical history, surgeries, etc.
- [ ] LAST—last intake & last output
- [ ] EVENT—events leading up to this crisis

SOAPNOTE—RECORD VITAL INFORMATION: ON-GOING ASSESSMENT

- [ ] Record patient data.
- [ ] Re-SOAP every 15 minutes.

MAKE A RESCUE PLAN

WILDERNESS FIRST AID

Part 4: STOP—Rescue Survey—how to get help

The Patient Assessment System has been completed. You now combine the patient's condition with the group's condition and determine if you need help from rescuers.

Patient's condition:
- Continuously monitor the patient's condition.
- Re-**SOAP** every 15 minutes.
  - **S**: are they hungry, thirsty, in pain, need to go to the bathroom?
  - **O**: take and record a complete set of vital signs, check all splints and bandages for circulation.
  - **A**: is assessment the same?
  - **P**: is the plan the same?

Group's condition:
- How well is each individual in the group doing: hungry, thirsty, anxious?
- How well-prepared is the group to stay put and bivouac?

Decisions:
- Do you need to evacuate the patient or can you all go on?
- If evacuation is needed, send for help.
- While waiting for rescue—build a bivouac.

Sending for help:
- Send two to get help if possible.
- Send out a SOAPnote on the patient.
- Send out a list of the remaining group and how well-prepared they are to bivouac.
- Send out a map with your exact location and time marked on it.

While waiting for help to arrive:
- Keep spirits up, be positive, reassure, make sure everyone has something to do.
- Create light and warmth; build a fire, keep everyone warm and dry.
- Make yourselves big, easy to find.
- Continuously monitor your patient and the other members of your group.

RESPONSE AND ASSESSMENT

PATIENT LIFTING & MOVING TECHNIQUES

When an injury occurs, it is important to keep the wounded person lying still, as they may not know how seriously they are hurt.

The very first component of patient care you will need to provide is to safely lift or move the patient to another location. This is to protect them from further harm or protect them from the environment. This may occur anytime during the Initial Assessment, Primary Survey, or Secondary Survey.

 Are they in immediate danger from rock fall, ice fall, avalanche, etc.?

 Are they lying in water?

 Are they lying on frozen ground or snow?

 Are they lying on sharp jagged rocks or other debris?

 Are they generally in harm's way?

If your patient is in harm's way, you are also in harm's way. One victim is enough.

When possible, try to perform a patient exam or chunk check before moving your patient so you have an idea of what the injuries are.

Personal Safety Precautions:

 Know your own strength and physical limitations.

 Work together—get as many hands on the patient as possible; many hands make light work.

31

The cardinal rule of moving hurt people...
It is always safe to move someone from the position of injury to the position of function.

...but
Avoid flexion of the head and neck.
- May move the head & neck into neutral position, but do not flex forward.

Avoid rotation of the pelvis out of alignment with the shoulders.
- May line up the shoulders and the pelvis, but do not rotate out of alignment.

POSITIONS:

SUPINE: Lying flat on your back.

PRONE: Lying flat on your chest & stomach.

RECOVERY POSITION: 3/4 prone position used to maintain the airway.

The recovery position.

When lifting, use proper body mechanics:

- Lift with your legs.
- Keep your back straight and your butt down.
- Try not to overreach or twist.
- Keep the weight as close to your body as possible.
- Use assists such as blankets, rain flies, or ensolite pads.

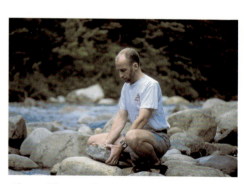
Always lift properly.

RESPONSE AND ASSESSMENT

LIFTING AND MOVING:

LOG ROLL: Keeping the head, shoulders, and pelvis in line, roll the patient onto their side.

MOVE AS A UNIT: With many hands on, move the person as if they were frozen stiff.

DRAGS: Drag them by their clothing or on a pad.

TRANSFERS & CARRIES: *With many hands, pick them up and walk:*

ONE-PERSON: Roll onto a pad to drag.

TWO-PERSON: May be able to carry or drag.

MANY PERSONS: Much easier, many hands on.

SHOCK

A condition in which the cardiovascular system fails to provide sufficient circulation to every part of the body causing tissues to eventually suffer from a lack of oxygen.

The CARDIOVASCULAR SYSTEM consists of:
- Heart—pumps the blood.
- Blood vessels—carry and distribute the blood.
- Blood—carries the oxygen.

Shock is a compensatory mechanism designed to keep the brain well-oxygenated during times of cardiovascular insufficiency by:
- Vasoconstricting the peripheral circulation, thus pooling blood into the body core,
- Increasing the heart rate, which sends more blood to the brain, and
- Increasing respiratory rate to maximize the amount of oxygen in the blood.

- These COMPENSATORY MECHANISMS occur whenever the BRAIN perceives a threat or crisis, real or not, and puts the cardiovascular system on ALERT STATUS. The ALERT STATUS is transient and self-correcting. SHOCK is the compensatory mechanism caused by failure of the cardiovascular system in its effort to maintain circulation and thus oxygen to the brain.
- In SHOCK the compensatory mechanism prioritizes the blood flow from the heart to the lungs to the brain. The only other organs involved are the liver and kidneys.
- Once injuries are properly treated, the shock condition or Alert Status should cease and the vital signs return to normal. If not, the person is in life-threatening shock.
- Initially shock status is a life-saving condition that preserves blood flow to the brain, but SHOCK KILLS if it continues for too long. You have to find the underlying cause.

Causes of shock:
- HYPOVOLEMIC: **LOW VOLUME** caused by decreased blood volume due to blood loss or dehydration from sweating, diarrhea, vomiting, or a burn.
- CARDIOGENIC: **LOW FLOW** caused by pump failure, i.e. a heart attack.
- NEUROGENIC: **LOW PRESSURE** caused by vasodilation, a loss of vascular tone, that results in increased vascular space, from spinal cord injury and acute allergic reaction to life-threatening infection, "blood poisoning," or septic shock.

RESPONSE AND ASSESSMENT

SIGNS & SYMPTOMS

Individuals in shock are not quite "there."

- They are distant.
- They stare off into space or may be unconscious.
- They may not know you are there.
- They may not feel pain or respond to pain.
- They may have an obvious wound or injury that they ignore.
- They may try to walk on a broken leg or use a broken arm.
- They do not know how seriously they are injured.
- They may have a sense of impending doom.

- LOC: restless, anxious, may be disoriented,
- RR: rapid & shallow (increased respiratory rate, more oxygen),
- HR: rapid & weak & thready (increased heart rate, to deliver more blood to the brain),
- SKIN: pale, cool, clammy (due to the vasoconstriction of the capillaries in the skin),
- May collapse; typically nauseous and may vomit.

CARE & TREATMENT:

- ✓ **AIRWAY, AIRWAY, AIRWAY.**
- ✓ Control **BLEEDING** to minimize blood loss.
- ✓ **FIND AND TREAT THE UNDERLYING CAUSE.**
- ✓ Treat all injuries to minimize pain.
- ✓ Keep them lying flat in a position of comfort; may elevate the legs.
- ✓ Protect from the environment; maintain body temperature.
- ✓ Monitor vital signs, reassure, & get help.

NOTES

CHAPTER TWO

TRAUMA: MUSCULOSKELETAL INJURIES
Strains, Sprains, and Fractures

TRAUMA: MUSCULOSKELETAL INJURIES

MUSCULOSKELETAL SYSTEM (BONES, MUSCLES, TENDONS, LIGAMENTS)

When your musculoskeletal system is working properly, this framework of bones, muscles, tendons, ligaments, and cartilage is what holds you up and allows you to move and function.

WHAT THEY DO:

- **BONES** provide the structure to which everything attaches. Bones also store calcium and produce blood cells in the bone marrow.

- **CARTILAGE** acts as a lubricated pad between bones so that your joints can flex or rotate smoothly. Cartilage also provides support for muscle in areas where more flexibility than bone is needed (like your ears).

- **SYNOVIAL FLUID** is the lubricant in the joint space and is produced by the synovial lining of the joint capsule.

- **MUSCLES** are like bundles of bungee cords. They contract or relax in response to signals sent from your brain through your central nervous system, which flexes your joints and allows you to move. Muscles also provide some padding and protection for nerve-bundles, arteries, and veins.

- **LIGAMENTS** are like nylon cords and attach bones to other bones. They maintain proper range of motion.

- **TENDONS** are ties connecting muscle to bone. They span joints and allow for movement.

TRAUMA: MUSCULOSKELETAL INJURIES

MUSCULOSKELETAL SYSTEM FUNCTIONS:

- Movement.
- Protection of underlying structures.
- Calcium storage.
- Blood cell production (Hematopoiesis).
- Heat production.
- Cosmesis (your muscles and bones determine how you look).

ANATOMICAL POSITION

When describing the position of parts of the body in relationship to each other, parts that are farther away from the core of the body are described as "DISTAL" and parts that are closer to the core of the body are "PROXIMAL."

TYPES OF MUSCULOSKELETAL INJURIES:

- Sprains and Strains—twisting and pulling damage to the supporting structure of joints (ligaments, muscles, and tendons) are by far the most common backcountry injuries.
- Fractures—breaks of the hard outer layer of bone can be particularly dangerous because the sharp ends of the bones can cause damage to the surrounding muscle, nerves, and blood vessels.

SPRAINS & STRAINS:

Signs and Symptoms:

- ✔ Generalized pain around a joint, no point tenderness.
- ✔ Pain with movement of the joint.
- ✔ Minimal pain with weight-bearing.
- ✔ Swelling can be dramatic.
- ✔ May become discolored over time, "black and blue" (ecchymosis).

Treatment: the primary goal is to minimize swelling by using RICE:

- ✔ Rest: stop and sit down; this slows circulation.
- ✔ Ice: causes vasoconstriction, decreasing circulation—ice, snow, or wet.
- ✔ Compression: decreases circulation and room for swelling; the less it swells the faster it will heal.
- ✔ Elevation: decreases circulation.
- ✔ Immobilize & support the affected joint.

TRAUMA: MUSCULOSKELETAL INJURIES

FRACTURES:
- Bones are made up of a hard outer layer of compact bone and an inner soft area of bone marrow.
- A fracture occurs when enough force is exerted against a bone to break the outer compact bone.

EVALUATING A MUSCULOSKELETAL INJURY:

	SPRAIN	FRACTURE
Look—What do you see when you examine the injury?		
Do they have normal movement and function?	Usually	No
Are they guarding the injury?	Slightly	Yes
Do you see any deformity or angulations?	No	Yes
Do you see any discoloration or swelling?	Maybe	Yes
Listen—Talk to the patient; what do they say?		
What happened?		
What was the Mechanism Of Injury (MOI)?		
Where does it hurt?		
Did they feel anything snap, crack, or pop?	Maybe	Usually
Feel—What do you feel when you examine the injury?		
Is there good Circulation, Sensation, and Motion (CSM)?	Usually	Maybe
Is there point tenderness?	No	Yes
Is there crepitation (the sound of broken bones grinding)?	No	Yes

Muscle under normal tension   Fracture

If the Mechanism of Injury indicates a possible fracture, treat as such.
WHEN IN DOUBT, SPLINT!
THE PRINCIPLES OF SPLINTING:

 Can the injury be immobilized in the position found? **Check circulation**.

 If not, pull **traction-in-line** to slowly and gently move the extremity into proper anatomical alignment. This establishes and maintains circulation distal to the site of the injury.

 Create a rigid but **well-padded** splint (well-insulated in winter); fill all voids.

 Immobilize the **entire extremity**, including the joint above and below the site of the injury.

 Monitor all splints; check C/S/M distal to the site of the injury every fifteen minutes.

SPLINTING PROCEDURES:

Improvise cervical collar:
- Used to protect neck.
- Soft, conforms to neck.
- Warm.
- Comfortable.

Arm sling & swathe—uses:
- Dislocated shoulder.
- Fractured clavicle.
- Fractured humerus.
- Fractured forearm, wrist, hand.
- Elbow injury.
- Fractured ribs.

TRAUMA: MUSCULOSKELETAL INJURIES

Forearm splint:
- Rigid splint with sticks, pack stays, etc. used with arm sling and swathe.
- Sam Splint used with arm sling and swathe.

Improvised lower leg & ankle splint:
- Rigid splint with sticks, poles, skis, etc.
- Ensolite pad splint.

Improvised knee splint:
- Splint knee in position of comfort (30° +/-).
- Place padding in the hollow behind the knee.

Sprained ankle bandage:
- To splint a fractured ankle or support a sprained ankle.

SPINAL CORD INJURY MANAGEMENT:

- Pre-hospital personnel are trained to treat all possible spinal cord injuries based on the Mechanism Of Injury (MOI) as well as symptoms and complaints.
- It is important in the wild environment for rescuers to recognize a possible back injury based on MOI, but it is equally important that they be able to rule it out or "clear the spine" by a proper history and physical exam in order to avoid an unnecessary litter evacuation.
- Spinal assessment—to clear the spine—is not performed until after the patient assessment system has been completed and it is appropriate to evaluate and potentially clear the spine of any possible injury.

Method of clearing the spine: Patient must meet all of these criteria to clear the spine.

- Patient must be sober, conscious, coherent, and oriented x 3, in person, place, & time.
- Patient has no painful distracting injuries (e.g. fractured femur, compound fracture, burn).
- Patient does not complain of any pain the entire length of the back.
- Patient does not have radiating pain, paresthesias (tingling), paralysis, or numbness in any of their extremities.
- Patient has intact sensation and motion in all four extremities unless local injury.
- Patient has no tenderness on physical exam along the entire length of the back.
- Without assistance, the patient is able to flex, extend, and rotate neck, upper, and lower back without pain or discomfort, and this movement is symmetrical without locking sensation or limited range of motion.
- You can always move the patient into proper anatomical position.

44

TRAUMA: MUSCULOSKELETAL INJURIES

SPINAL CORD INJURY MANAGEMENT:

- It is more important to know how to move an injured person, to protect them from further injury than it is to know how to backboard them.
- Cervical spine is at risk with flexion; do not lift head.
- Lumbar spine is at risk with rotation; keep shoulders, and hips aligned.
- Lifting and moving techniques were discussed with Patient Assessment.

Cervical Collars:

- You can improvise very comfortable and immobilizing soft blanket and horseshoe collars out of materials such as a pile jacket, blanket, or ensolite pad. They provide support, comfort, and warmth.

Backboards:

- Backboards or litters are only used by rescue teams for transport.
- While waiting for help to arrive, simply keep the patient still, comfortable, and warm.
- Protect them from the cold or hot ground.
- Remember not to flex the neck! Keep the spine straight by log rolling the patient.

45

NOTES

CHAPTER THREE

ENVIRONMENTAL EMERGENCIES & SURVIVAL SKILLS

How To Survive and Thrive in the World

ENVIRONMENTAL EMERGENCIES AND SURVIVAL SKILLS:

Before you examine environmental threats, it is critical that you understand how your body reacts to changes in your environment. You have characteristics that make you both wonderfully suited to your environment and yet terribly susceptible to its fluctuations.

THE HUMAN ANIMAL

- Humans are a true tropical animal—an essentially hairless being with sweat glands.
- You are warm-blooded and, through metabolism, are constantly generating heat.
- Your skin is your largest organ, accounting for about 10% of your body's weight; it is the primary organ of thermoregulation.
- You have one of the most sensitive and efficient regulatory mechanisms on the planet for surviving and thriving in the heat; it is designed to keep your brain at a relatively constant temperature.
- You sweat, and the evaporation of water from your skin cools the blood in the skin and, thus, the systemic circulation. Fur-covered mammals and birds pant, which evaporates water out of the airways, thus cooling their blood in the pulmonary circulation.
- You do not survive because of physical prowess but by your mental prowess.
- You have only rudimentary defensive mechanisms to protect you in the cold (e.g. frostbite only numbs us; it does not produce a painful warning).

Because of these characteristics, humans are perfectly suited to life in the tropics where the ability to shed heat is more important than the ability to retain it. However, as populations grew and moved north or south of the tropics, this ability became a hinderance because they often found themselves cooling off faster than they could generate or maintain heat, resulting in hypothermia, risk of frostbite, and impaired mental function. "A cold brain is a dumb brain."

ENVIRONMENTAL EMERGENCIES & SURVIVAL SKILLS

THE HUMAN BRAIN

- In order for your brain to function normally, it needs a constant supply of oxygen and glucose, and a consistent temperature between 97^0 and 104^0F.
- Anatomy and Function: You can think of the brain like an onion with each layer that is added on being a layer of increased function or intelligence.
- The **Brainstem** is at the top of the spinal cord in the center of the brain. It controls the functions that maintain life from second-to-second ("reptilian brain"). Found in this structure are:
    - The respiratory center that controls breathing.
    - The cardiovascular center that controls heart rate and blood pressure.
    - The thermoregulatory center that maintains core temperature.
    - The reticuloactivating center that maintains level of consciousness.
- The **Primitive Brain** or **limbic brain** surrounds the brainstem. It controls the functions that allow you to survive day-to-day and as a species ("primitive brain"):
    - The need to procreate (sex drive).
    - Defensive posturing, primitive aggressive reflexes.
- The **Higher Brain** or **cerebral cortex** is what makes you human. It controls the functions that allow you to survive, strive, and thrive:
    - Gross motor coordination.
    - Fine motor coordination.
    - Reasoning, problem-solving, and judgment.
- When you impair the brain, it loses functions from the most advanced layer, the outermost layer, in. So you lose judgment and problem-solving first and the ability to breathe last.

THERMOREGULATION: BALANCING THE TEMPERATURE

HEAT PRODUCTION:
- Basal metabolism is the constant biochemistry that produces heat.
- You burn glucose to produce the heat to drive other chemical reactions.
- Exercise, muscle activity, produces heat.
- Voluntary or involuntary shivering can increase heat production 5x's.

HEAT CONSERVATION:
- Vasoconstriction of the blood vessels in the skin.
- Piloerection—hair standing on end.
- Cessation of sweating.
- Posturing—assuming positions to conserve body heat.

PHYSICS OF HEAT LOSS: (LAWS OF THERMODYNAMICS):
- Conduction   0%–40% depending upon the type of solid material.
- Convection   0%–40% depending upon air penetration.
- Radiation   5%–80% depending upon surrounding temperature.
- Evaporation   0%–90% depending upon vapor pressure & moisture.

conduction

radiation

convection

evaporation

ENVIRONMENTAL EMERGENCIES & SURVIVAL SKILLS

NUTRITION:

Nutritional Requirements: the average person needs about 2500 calories/day.
- Carbohydrate: 4cal/gram   60%   (200–400 grams/day = 1200–1600 cal/day).
- Protein: 4cal/gram   30%   (30–55 grams/day = 120–220 cal/day).
- Fat: 9cal/gram   10%   (20–60 grams/day = 180–540 cal/day).

Number of calories required varies with activity:
- Normal daily activity: 2000–2500 calories/day.
- Winter outdoor sports: 3000–4000 calories/day.
- High altitude activities: 4000–6000 calories/day.

HYDRATION:

Hydration Requirements: the average person needs about two liters of fluid per day.

Normal water losses per day:	Normal Temp	Hot Temp	Heavy Exercise
Skin (moisture loss)	350ml	350ml	350ml
Respiration (breathing)	250ml	350ml	650ml
Sweating	100ml	1400ml	**5000ml**
Urination	1400ml	1200ml	500ml
Defecation	100ml	100ml	100ml
TOTALS	**2200ml**	**3400ml**	**6600ml**

Water requirements will vary with activity, sweat output, and altitude.
- Exertional sweat loss is 1–3 liters/hour for up to 4 hours without replacement.
- Altitude has a very low vapor pressure; you will lose about 1cup/hour via respirations.
  (24 cups/24 hrs., 6 quarts or liters/24 hrs., 1½ gallons every 24 hrs.)

You have to be able to make pure potable (drinkable) water.
- If you have to melt snow, you have to know how much fuel to carry.
- Potable water—chemicals, filtering, boiling.

Altitude: we are designed to live between sea level and 8000 feet.
- 8000–14000 feet—the upper limits of sustainable life.
- 14000–18000 feet—high altitude you can visit.
- 18000–28000 feet—very high altitude, constant negative deficit.
- Risk of altitude illness can occur above 5000 feet.
- Risk is increased by rate of ascent. Safe ascent is 1000 feet/day.
- Risk is increased by dehydration, exhaustion, and alcohol consumption.

HYPOTHERMIA:

Hypothermia: Is a lowering of the body's core temperature to a level where normal brain & muscle function are impaired. Remember the onion analogy. As the body cools, function is lost from the most advanced layer down.

- Lizard—reptilian (rudimentary) brain
- Lemur—limbic (primitive) brain
- Human—cortex (higher) brain

- People suffering from hypothermia do "mindless" things like leaving food, water, and shelter behind.
- Hypothermia is insidious in that you cannot detect the danger signs in yourself.
- Even though the signs and symptoms of hypothermia may be very obvious when exhibited in others, when you become hypothermic, you think everything is fine.

The body's defensive reaction to cooling off: Losing more heat than it produces.

- Skin: peripheral vasoconstriction to decrease blood flow to the skin and thus decrease heat loss.
- Involuntary shivering: uncoordinated muscle activity to produce heat.
- Increased basal metabolism: burn glucose to produce heat—rate may increase 5 fold.
- Behavioral: put on warm clothes, seek out shelter, warmth, protection.

There is no warning of impending doom:

- You do not have a cold center in your brain that warns you that you are becoming hypothermic.
- You get cold, you get dumb, you get lost, you get hurt, you cause problems.

Stages of Hypothermia:

- 98.6F Normal
- 97F   The brain falters, judgment fails, protective & survival instincts decrease. At this point you are in trouble, as you do not take measures to protect yourself. As temperature decreases, mental abilities decrease.
- 96F   Shivering begins, a constant fine motor tremor. You cannot stop it. It interferes with coordinated muscle activity.
- 94F   You shiver harder; coordination is failing; you begin tripping and falling.
- 92F   Shivering is intense; you are unable to walk.
- 90F   Shivering is convulsive; you assume the fetal position; you are unable to talk.
- 86F   and below: The "Metabolic Icebox;" you are unconscious, ashen gray; you may appear pulseless and breathless.

ENVIRONMENTAL EMERGENCIES & SURVIVAL SKILLS

Prevention: Know your enemy and be prepared for wet, wind, & cold.

- ✔ Carry and use rain gear: pants and jacket.
- ✔ Wear fabrics that stay warm when wet.
- ✔ Snack often on foods high in quick-burning carbohydrates/glucose.
- ✔ Stay WELL-HYDRATED.
- ✔ Carry bivouac gear and know how to use it.
- ✔ Be attentive to yourself, companions and the environment.

Treatment: Remove the patient from immediate danger & further exposure.

- ✔ Create or seek out shelter.
- ✔ Get DRY & keep DRY.
- ✔ Give lots of warm, sweet liquids (JELL-O with <u>sugar</u>) if conscious.
- ✔ Insulate with hypothermia wrap.

 The preferred method for field rewarming of a hypothermic patient involves two principles: Helping the patient to continue to generate body heat and preventing the patient from losing that heat to the environment.

 One of the best ways to generate body heat is to feed fuel to the furnace. Foods like powdered JELL-O dissolved in warm water are easy for most patients to take and can provide the needed caloric energy for the patient to start generating more heat.

53

HYPOTHERMIA: THE HYPOWRAP— BUILDING THE HUMAN BURRITO

Once refueling has started, the next step is to stop the patient from losing body heat and create an environment that allows them to store the heat they are producing. The Hypowrap provides an excellent environment for rewarming and protects the patient from the weather.

- Get the patient dry and keep them dry.
- Remove any wet clothing from the patient.
- Reinsulate them with **DRY MATERIAL**—clothing, sleeping bags.
- Place them on an insulating layer such as a dry foam pad.
- Surround the patient with a windproof, waterproof layer—plastic sheeting, tarp.
- Monitor their condition and take appropriate actions as conditions change.

PRINCIPLES OF TREATING HYPOTHERMIA

- Protect from the environment.
- Stop the heat loss.
- Stoke the fire—feed and hydrate.
- Insulate to minimize heat loss.
- If unconscious, do not attempt to feed.
- Make sure everyone in the group is warm and dry.

ENVIRONMENTAL EMERGENCIES & SURVIVAL SKILLS

Prepare a base of protective and insulating material. Windproof and waterproof outer layer with insulating layer (ensolite).

Add lots of dry insulation.

Place patient inside. Double-protect feet and head.

Wrap securely and monitor condition.

FROSTBITE:

Frostbite: Is a localized cooling and/or freezing of tissue caused by the shunting of blood away from cold areas of the body.

Superficial: description and treatment:
- 1st degree: "frostnip"—numb, soft, cold, pallor.
- 2nd degree: numb, soft, cold, pallor, pain on thawing, and formation of clear fluid-filled or blood-filled bleb.
- Field rewarm using skin-to-skin contact.
- Never massage, rub with snow, or use an external heat source.
- If a bleb forms, protect the area and evacuate the patient.
- Beware of refreezing which can happen quickly and will cause much greater tissue damage.

Deep: description and treatment:
- 3rd degree: numb, cold, white, and rock hard; massive blebs form when thawed; extreme pain during thawing.
- Protect the area and evacuate the patient.
- DO NOT field rewarm (once thawed the area is useless and excruciatingly painful).

1st degree

2nd degree with bleb

3rd degree

ENVIRONMENTAL EMERGENCIES & SURVIVAL SKILLS

Prevention: Keep the whole body warm.

- ✓ If your feet are cold, put on a hat.
- ✓ Eat & drink to maintain a constant energy/heat production—maintain blood sugar.
- ✓ STAY DRY! CARRY AND USE RAIN GEAR—TOPS & BOTTOMS.
- ✓ Pack extra socks, hats, mittens, or any clothing that is likely to get wet.
- ✓ Wear wool or pile. (Cotton is warm only as long as it is dry.)
- ✓ Do not drink alcohol or use tobacco.
- ✓ Avoid tight clothing, boots, crampons.
- ✓ Keep an eye on each other.

HEAT INJURIES:

Heat Exhaustion:
- Not a life-threatening emergency. Heat-exhausted patients often recover without care.
- Usually occurs in people who are not acclimatized to heat.
- Cause: A combination of salt and water loss secondary to sweating = dehydration.
- May be associated with heat cramps.
- Heat exhaustion can progress to heat stroke.

***Signs & Symptoms:** Typically complain of mild headache, dizziness, and nausea.*
- Skin: pale, cool, clammy.
- LOC: may be normal or slightly anxious.
- Pulse: slightly increased, but BP is normal.
- Resp.: may be normal or slightly increased with normal effort.

Treatment:
- Rest in a cool place in the shade.
- Replace lost fluid & salt—1 teaspoon salt + 8 teaspoons of sugar in 1 liter/quart of water. This is an oral rehydration solution (ORS). ORS can also be used to replace fluids lost from diarrhea, vomiting, fever (sweating), or burns. Other ORS are:
    - Commercial: Gatorade
    - Fruits: oranges, melons, lemons, and limes, either eaten or juiced

one teaspoon salt

plus eight teaspoons sugar

plus one liter water

EQUALS TREATMENT

ENVIRONMENTAL EMERGENCIES & SURVIVAL SKILLS

Heat Stroke:

A true LIFE-THREATENING EMERGENCY! The patient will die without immediate care!

Two Causes:
- One: The person has become dehydrated by sweating out fluid faster than they replace it. As their sweating mechanism fails, their body temperature goes up rapidly.
- Two: With a hot day and high humidity, the sweat cannot evaporate off their skin fast enough to cool them. (Exertional heatstroke).

Signs & Symptoms:
- Skin: RED, HOT, DRY (50%); OTHER 50% ARE WET.
- Temp.: $105°F+$, maximum survivable core temperature is $107°F$.
- LOC: Disoriented, confused, combative, hallucinating, eventually coma & death.
- Pulse: Rapid and full; BP may be elevated.
- Resp.: Full and deep.

Treatment: *This is one of the few conditions where immediate treatment is essential.*
- REMOVE FROM HEAT & SUN.
- COOL IMMEDIATELY by soaking with water & fanning to accelerate evaporation.
- Hydrate if possible.
- Vigorously massage limbs.
- Beware of shivering—shivering produces heat.
- Transport immediately to the hospital.

Prevention: *Stay out of the hot noonday sun.*
- Hydrate or die.
- Stay hydrated & eat salty foods.
- Keep your head covered; wear cotton that will hold moisture which cools the skin.
- Beware of warning signs: feel hot, feel dry, can't pee.

59

NORTH AMERICAN BITES AND STINGS

Three Primary Concerns:
- Tissue damage
- Envenomation
- Infection by microorganisms (viruses, bacteria, malaria, Lyme)

MAMMALS

Despite the unlikelihood of being bitten by a wild animal, there are some general things to remember that may help prevent a bite from occurring:
- Never attempt to approach or feed a wild animal; they're called wild for a reason.
- Keep a clean kitchen; bag and hang food; dispose of scraps/waste properly.
- Never tease or make aggressive movements toward wild animals.
- Bites may cause wounds: punctures, lacerations, avulsions.

Treatment:
- Stop the bleeding.
- Scrub the wound aggressively; try to move saliva out and away from the wound.
- Irrigate the wound generously with a dilute (1%) iodine solution.
- Do not close any animal bite in the field; the chance of infection is high.
- Is there a risk of rabies exposure? If so, consider rabies vaccine.

SNAKES
- The primary reason people are bitten by snakes is that they pick them up.
- Bites usually occur on the hand.

Poisonous snakes of North America:
- Pit Vipers (Viperidsd): They inject a hemotoxin that is meant to both poison and digest prey.
    - Rattlesnakes
    - Copperheads
    - Water Moccasins
- Coral Snake (Elapids): Small, shy, and timid, this snake has a very powerful neurotoxin; however, bites are rare, and deaths are rarer.

Treatment of snake bites:
DO'S
- ✓ DO CALL 911, seek immediate help
- ✓ DO KEEP THEM CALM, lay them down and keep them comfortable
- ✓ DO TRY TO ID THE SNAKE, but do not get bit, one patient is enough
- ✓ DO REMOVE ANY CONSTRICTING CLOTHING OR JEWELERY, the bite sitand the extremity will swell
- ✓ DO PLACE THE BITE SITE BELOW THE LEVEL OF THE HEART
- ✓ DO CONSIDER A PRESSURE IMMOBILIZATION WRAP, but not with a rattlesnake bites (pit vipers – Viperids)
- ✓ DO MONITOR YOUR PATIENT AND MONITOR FOR ANAPHYLAXIS

ENVIRONMENTAL EMERGENCIES & SURVIVAL SKILLS

DON'TS

- DO NOT USE TOURNIQUETS
- DO NOT CUT AND SUCK, do not make a "X" over the fang sites in an effort to suck out the venom
- DO NOT APPLY ICE
- DO NOT ELECTROCUTE, do not use a stun gun in an effort to destroy the venom with elecricity
- DO NOT GIVE ASPIRIN OR ANY OTHER NSAID
- DO NOT EXERT, in other words, do not let them exercise, no exertion
- DO NOT GIVE THEM ANY CAFFEINE OR OTHER STIMULANT
- DO NOT USE AN EXTRACTOR, to try to suck out the venom
- DO NOT HANDLE THE SNAKE, even if dead can still strike
- DO NOT CLEAN THE WOUND, may be able to ID the snake by the venom

PRESSURE IMMOBILIZATION WRAP:

Gently wrap the extremity that was bitten with a 4 – 6" elastic wrap.
Wrap distal to proximal with gently compression, enough to stop the lymphatic drainage, but not enough to impair circulation.
This technique is controversial, some feel that if used with pit vipers, a hemotoxin that also digest tissues, by isolating the venom, the gently compression wrap may increase the risk of further tissue damage.

INSECTS

- Hymenoptera: Bees, Hornets, Wasps, Fire Ants

Signs and Symptoms:
- Pain, local swelling, redness, and itching are common.

Treatment:
- Remove stinger/poison sack by scraping; do not use tweezers.
- Assess and Monitor for anaphylaxis.
- Use topical "bite and sting" stick for comfort.
- Give an oral antihistamine to prevent an allergic reaction: Benadryl (diphenhydramine) 25mg, 2 every 4 hours x 24 hours.

Ticks:

They are tiny septic tanks and carry several infectious diseases.
- Can spread Lyme Disease (the most common, but ticks can carry eight other diseases).
- Small to tiny with large abdomens and short legs.
- Color ranges from tan to brown, almost black.
- They attach to the host, bury their head in the skin, and take a blood meal for a day or more.
- Disease is spread by their saliva, an anticoagulant.

Treatment:
- Remove by pulling off (grasp as close to skin as possible); clean area well.

Mosquitoes and other blood-sucking insects:

- Can be vectors for infectious diseases: Malaria, Equine Enchephalitis, Nile Virus, etc.
- Avoid being bitten by using insect repellents, protective clothing, and sleeping under mosquito netting.

LIGHTNING

Laws of Nature:
- Lightning can and will do anything. It is unpredictable and uncontrollable.
- Lightning is most likely to strike the highest object around and follow the path of least resistance.

Rules to Live by:
- Thunderstorms are most dangerous as they approach, especially when within 1 mile.
- Don't be the highest object around to avoid a DIRECT STRIKE.
- Stay away from the highest objects to avoid SPLASH or STEP VOLTAGE.
- If on or near water, get off and away from the shoreline.
- Don't sit under overhangs or get into shallow caves.
- Lightning flows like water, so stay out of gullies and washes.
- Calculating Lightning's Distance—Light 286,000 miles/second vs. Sound 700 mph. Count the delay between flash and rumble: 5 seconds = 1 mile.
- Thunderstorms travel at approximately 20-25 mph, e.g. a storm approaching from 3 miles away (15 sec) will be in striking range in 6 minutes.

Places to Avoid or Get off:
- Mountain summits.
- Ridges and cliff tops.
- Overhangs and shallow caves.
- Ditches, gullies, streams.
- Tall trees, poles, large boulders, high objects.
- Open areas, fields, meadows, any place in which you are the highest object.

What to Do If Caught Out:

 Get off the summit and below tree line if possible.

 Once below treeline, seek out a low spot among small trees.

 Stay away from tall trees, cliff faces, and streams.

 Sit on your pack, pad, or other insulator with your knees flexed, and hug your knees.

 Keep your feet together to minimize the ground effect of a near-by strike.

ENVIRONMENTAL EMERGENCIES & SURVIVAL SKILLS

Injuries: May Include:
- Respiratory arrest that can progress to cardiac arrest.
- Burns.
- Soft Tissue Injuries.
- Musculoskeletal injuries.

Treatment:
- ✓ Maintain ABCs; closely monitor for respiratory arrest.
- ✓ Do a complete physical exam.
- ✓ Treat all injuries.
- ✓ If conscious, force fluids to help prevent late complications.
- ✓ Evacuate.

THE BACKCOUNTRY ESSENTIALS:

ATTITUDE: THINK POSITIVELY.
- Positive attitude: belief that you can always make things better.
- Will to survive.

FOOD: GET FUEL TO BURN.
- High carbohydrate foods that require no preparation & provide quick energy.
- High carbohydrate foods that can be made into a warm drink (Jello).

WATER: QUENCH YOUR THIRST.
- Minimum of 2 liters per day if not active (up to 1-3 liters/hour if active).
- The ability to disinfect water (chemicals, filtering, boiling).

CLOTHING: STAY WARM & DRY.
- Warm clothing that retains heat even when wet (spare socks & hat).
- Waterproof rain gear, both tops and bottoms (large garbage or leaf bags).

SHELTER: GET DRY & STAY DRY.
- Ability to improvise shelter (10' x 10' plastic sheet, p-cord, space blanket).
- Comfort & light (plumber's candles).

FIRE: GET WARM.
- Ability to build a fire (waterproof matches, tinder, candles).
- Ability to make kindling (pocket knife).
- Ability to warm water (tin cup).

ENVIRONMENTAL EMERGENCIES & SURVIVAL SKILLS

NAVIGATION: KNOW WHERE YOU'RE GOING.
- Map & Compass; know how to use them.
- Ability to find your way at night (route-finding skills and flashlight).

WEATHER: KNOW THE ENVIRONMENT.
- Basic understanding of weather patterns.
- Knowledge of how to react to severe weather, lightning, etc.

SIGNALING: GET HELP.
- Whistle (preferably plastic) and signal mirror (whistle and/or mirror).

EXPERIENCE: PRACTICE SURVIVAL SKILLS BEFORE YOU NEED THEM.
- The most valuable and versatile survival tool is between your ears.

AVOID THE SURVIVAL SITUATION:

 Make a plan and work the plan.

 Know your limitations and the group's limitations.

65

BIVUOAC & SURVIVAL SKILLS:

CRISIS INTERVENTION:

- Be prepared to bivouac.
- Keep everyone warm and dry.
- Know how to get help.
- Send out two for help.
- Send out a SOAPnote.
    - Send out your group's ability to stay put.
    - Send out a map with your exact location marked on it.
    - Know how to build a fire and make yourself very big, easy to find (surveyor's tape).

Factors that contribute to a crisis:

- Fatigue, taking on too much.
- Pushing hard or rushing to get someplace.
- Weather.
- Equipment failure or, more often, the wrong equipment.
- Lack of equipment.
- Personality problems.
- Poor judgment, making wrong decisions for wrong reasons—ego.

IF YOU WANT TO BE FOUND:

 "Hug a tree" - Stay put, don't wander around.

 Make yourself big and obvious:
- Build a smoky fire.
- Put out long pieces of brightly colored surveyor's tape.
- Mark the area with broken branches, clothing.

BIVOUAC KIT: THE 16 ESSENTIALS FOR YOUR BACKPACK:

Best option—Carry a "bivy kit" in a stuff sack:
- Spare hat—balaclava; can cover your whole face and neck.
- Spare socks—for feet and can also act as emergency mittens.
- Space blanket or big garbage/leaf bag.
- Metal cup—that you can hold over a candle or fire to melt snow.
- JELL-O—with real sugar.
- Hard candies—with real sugar.
- Plumber's candles—short, thick, and long-burning.
- Waterproof matches—some people like to also carry a lighter.
- Compass.
- Whistle and/or signaling mirror.
- Knife.
- Parachute cord—100".
- Surveyor's tape—bright color.
- Plastic 6 mil or tarp—10' x 10'.
- Paper and pencil.
- Duct tape.

Bivouac Skills: What to do with what you have:

Improvised shelters—bivouacs:
- Severe weather bivouac—"bombproof."
- Lean-to—roomy, but easily blown apart.
- Worst option: Just you, "WHAT IF!" NO FOOD, NO WATER, NO SHELTER?

No snow—debris piles:
- Large overhanging trees.
- Overhangs & caves.

Snow—snow piles = Quinzee:
- Snow trenches.
- Snow caves.
- Large evergreens with branches close to the ground.

— *NOTES*—

CHAPTER FOUR

SOFT TISSUE INJURIES & MEDICAL EMERGENCIES
From Minor Wounds to Critical Care

SOFT TISSUE INJURIES:

SOFT TISSUES:
- Everything except the bones.
- This section concentrates on insults and injuries to the skin and structures immediately under the skin: fat, muscles, & blood vessels.

Remember: Total Body Fluid Precautions—BSI

THE PIPES: ARTERIES, VEINS, & CAPILLARIES

They are muscular tubes that expand and contract depending on required blood flow.
- Arteries are the blood vessels leaving the heart.
    - They are under pressure: the systolic blood pressure—100 to 120 mmHg
    - Arteries are deep, protected, lying under the muscles directly on top of the bones.
    - When arteries are cut, they spurt like little oil wells—this is very rare.
- Veins are the blood vessels returning to the heart.
    - They are under very little pressure—10 to 20 mmHg pressure.
    - Veins are superficial and can be seen and felt under the skin.
    - When veins are cut, they drain blood. How much depends on the diameter of the vein.
- Capillaries are the tiny blood vessels that carry oxygen to the cells.
    - They are microscopic.
    - They are the most abundant vessels in the body.
    - One pound of body tissue has 1 mile of capillaries.
    - Capillaries in the skin expand and contract to control blood flow to the skin.
    - When cut, they seep or ooze blood

THE LIQUID: BLOOD—"THE RED STUFF"
- Carries oxygen, nutrients, and water to all the cells of the body.
- Carries away carbon dioxide and waste products.
- Carries heat into the extremities.
- Loss of blood causes a potentially life-threatening condition—SHOCK.

SOFT TISSUE INJURIES & MEDICAL EMERGENCIES

PRINCIPLES OF MANAGING SOFT TISSUE INJURIES:
- Control Bleeding
- Clean
- Bandage
- Monitor

TO CONTROL BLEEDING:

✓ Direct Pressure:
- Apply pressure directly over the wound and compress to stop the bleeding.
- Maintain pressure for about 10 minutes.

✓ Elevation:
- Along with direct pressure you can elevate the wound above the heart to decrease the pressure in the vessel, making it easier to stop the bleeding.

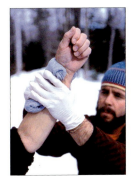

✓ Pressure Dressing:
- To maintain constant pressure, place something bulky and absorbent over the wound, an inch or two thick.
- Wrap the dressing with an elastic bandage for about 10 minutes.
- Then loosen the dressing to ensure circulation distal to the injury.
- Once bleeding has been controlled for 20–30 minutes, direct pressure can be stopped so the wound can be inspected and properly cleaned.

BUT WHAT IF...

✓ If unable to control bleeding with direct pressure and elevation:
- Remove the dressings and inspect the wound—you will find a spurting artery.
- Apply digital pressure with a finger to the little bleeder and hold pressure for ten minutes. (BSI!)
- Consider hemostatic agent
- Consider tourniquet

71

SPECIFIC SOFT TISSUE INJURIES:

Contusions:
- Bruises: mild swelling, discoloration, may be painful.

 Rest, Ice, Compression, and Elevation (RICE) to limit swelling.

 Protect and watch injury closely in cold weather as it will freeze quicker than usual.

Abrasions:
- Scrapes may be painful, dirty, and can easily become infected.

 Very little bleeding; while wound is pain-free, scrub thoroughly with soap & water.

 Allow to air dry before bandaging.

 You may apply antibiotic ointment for comfort.

Lacerations/Incisions:
- May bleed profusely or require pressure dressing.

 Control bleeding and maintain hemostasis for 20–30 minutes.

 Cleanse well with copious irrigation.

 For large gaping wound—control bleeding, cleanse, approximate edges, don't close tightly.

 If stitched or butterflied closed, infection is likely. It may have to be re-opened.

Flap Avulsion:
- Three-sided tear, one side still attached.

 Control bleeding; then rinse under flap with water, and bandage it in its anatomical position.

SOFT TISSUE INJURIES & MEDICAL EMERGENCIES

Amputation:
- A body part is completely severed.
  - Wrap the part in a moist sterile dressing, and seal it in a plastic bag.
  - Immerse the bag in ice water, and evacuate both the patient and the part to the hospital.

Punctures:
- Small penetrating wound to the skin.
  - Gently irritate to cause some bleeding to flush out the wound.
  - Monitor for infection; this is the wound most likely to become infected.

Impaled Objects:
- Something stuck in the body that doesn't belong there.
  - Use common sense; if easily removed, remove it.
  - Once removed, use direct pressure to control bleeding..

- Impaled object may be removed if:
  - It is in an extremity.
  - It is in the cheek of the face (or buttocks).
  - It is metal in a cold environment.
  - It is too large or hard to cut off.

- Do not remove impaled objects if: (These objects should be bandaged in place.)
  - In the skull or neck.
  - In the chest, possibly into the lungs.
  - In the abdomen, possibly penetrating.

- What about fish hooks?
  - Easily removed by pushing away from the barb and backing out.

73

SOFT TISSUE INJURIES:

LONG-TERM WOUND CARE—DEFINITIVE CARE IS LONGER THAN 24 HOURS AWAY:

Prevent infection and promote healing by:

- Properly cleaning the wound—once bleeding has been controlled for 20-30 minutes:

  - ✓ Remove dressings and closely inspect the wound.
  - ✓ Check circulation, sensation, and motion (CSM) distal to the injury.
  - ✓ Debride, remove any foreign material in the wound like sticks, grass, etc.
  - ✓ Clean around the wound with soap & water or with a dilute solution of iodine.
  - ✓ Clean the wound by irrigation with a forceful flow of sterile water or a dilute solution of iodine by using an irrigation syringe or water bottle.
  - ✓ Cover the wound with dry sterile dressings and keep clean & dry.
  - ✓ Bandage the sterile dressings in place.
  - ✓ Change the dressings every 12 hours, and examine the wound for signs of infection.

But what if...

- If the wound is dirty or unable to be kept clean and dry:

  - ✓ Cover the wound with a dressing soaked with a dilute solution of iodine, less than 2% strength.
  - ✓ Change every 6 hours.

- There is impaired CSM distal to the injury:

  - ✓ Do all of the above.
  - ✓ Then splint.
  - ✓ Then evacuate.

SOFT TISSUE INJURIES & MEDICAL EMERGENCIES

WOUND CARE DO'S AND DON'TS:

DO'S

 Protect from further injury, freezing, and from contamination by proper bandaging.

DON'TS

 Don't tightly close a wound with butterfly bandages or suturing.

 Don't fill the wound with an antibiotic ointment.

 Don't leave a pressure dressing in place for more than 20 minutes.

 Don't allow the wound to freeze.

 Don't be afraid of causing pain to properly clean a wound.

INFECTIONS:

- Caused by contamination of the wound by bacteria.
- Bacteria want to be warm, moist, and in the dark.
- Bacteria double (reproduce) every 30 minutes at 98^0F (37^0C).
- Signs and symptoms of an infection are a result of your immune system's response to the invading bacteria.
- Risk of tetanus; know shot status (good for ten years).

FECUNDITY GONE AWRY

No. of Bacteria	Elapsed Hours	
1	0	—
16	2	tens
256	4	hundreds
1,024	5	thousands
131,072	8.5	hundreds of thousands
1,048,376	10	millions
1,073,537,024	15	billions
1,024,000,000,000	20	trillions
256,000,000,000,000	24	256 trillion hungry little mouths to feed

Signs of infection:

Early: localized to the skin and wound area:
- Red (rubor)—due to dilated capillary beds, increased blood flow to the area.
- Warm (calor)—due to the increased blood flow.
- Swollen (tumor)—due to the increased blood flow.
- Tender (dolor)—due to swelling.

Late—severe potentially life-threatening:
- Pus formation—collection of white blood cells, may be draining from the wound.
- Streaking up the extremity—due to infection traveling up lymphatics.
- Swollen and tender lymph nodes—the infection has reached the lymph nodes.
- Fever and Chills—a sign that the infection is spreading systemically, septic shock.

Treatment of skin infections:

✓ Apply moist heat packs; if possible, soak in hot water with salt.

✓ If the wound is closed but swollen, gently open so it can drain.

✓ Evacuate as soon as possible if red streaks and/or fever develop.

WHEN SHOULD YOU EVACUATE FOR STITCHES?

- If the cut goes through the skin (causes gaping) and is longer than 1 inch—cosmetic repair.
- If the cut is in the face, hands, or over a joint.
- If there is an injury to a nerve, ligament, or tendon.

SOFT TISSUE INJURIES & MEDICAL EMERGENCIES

- Check for distal CIRCULATION, SENSATION, and MOTION.

THERMAL BURNS

Treatment: get the heat out:

- ✔ Remove clothing over and around the burn site.
- ✔ Cool with cold water for at least 15 minutes.

Superficial: First & Second Degree Burns:

- Appearance: area of the burn will turn red and may form blisters, but the patient has full sensation.
  - ✔ Cold soak the burn with water for 15 minutes.
  - ✔ Protect with a moist sterile dressing.
  - ✔ Evacuate if the burn area is more than the size of their palm.
  - ✔ If the burn area is large and painful, cover with moist dressings for comfort during evacuation.

Deep: Third Degree

- Appearance: area of the burn may be red, white, charred, blistered, but there is no sensation; the burn is deep enough to destroy the sensory nerves.
  - ✔ All deep burns must be evacuated.
  - ✔ Cold soak the burn with water for 15 minutes.
  - ✔ Cover with a moist dressing and waterproof bandage to prevent evaporation.
  - ✔ Hydrate—force fluids as burns can cause severe dehydration.

BLISTERS:

- Caused by friction against the skin forcing the layers of the skin apart.
- Common causes are a loose boot or shoe rubbing against the heel, or a shovel handle or oar-loom rubbing against the palms of the hands.
- The body reacts to the abuse by secreting water into the area of trauma.
- Blisters start out as a "hot spot" that, if left unattended to, will grow into a water-filled blister or bleb.

Treatment:

- React to the pain or "hot spot."
  - ✔ If on the foot, remove the sock and boot and apply athletic tape over the hot spot.
  - ✔ Then redress the foot paying attention to how the sock and boot fit.

- If a fluid-filled blister has formed, properly treat and protect the blister.
  - ✔ Clean the area around the blister.
  - ✔ Drain the blister by making small holes around the base with a sterile needle, and gently compress the blister to force out the fluid.
  - ✔ Surround the blister with padding, moleskin, molefoam, Spenco Second Skin, etc.
  - ✔ Fill the well created by the blister dressing with an antibiotic ointment to protect the fragile skin and minimize friction.
  - ✔ Cover the blister area and padding with tape.
  - ✔ If on the foot, redress the foot.
  - ✔ Clean daily and monitor for signs of infection.

SOFT TISSUE INJURIES & MEDICAL EMERGENCIES

PREVENTION:

- Sock combination—thin on skin, thick over
- Properly fit boots—break them in
- React early to pain or hot spots
- Keep feet dry—wet feet blister easily and quickly

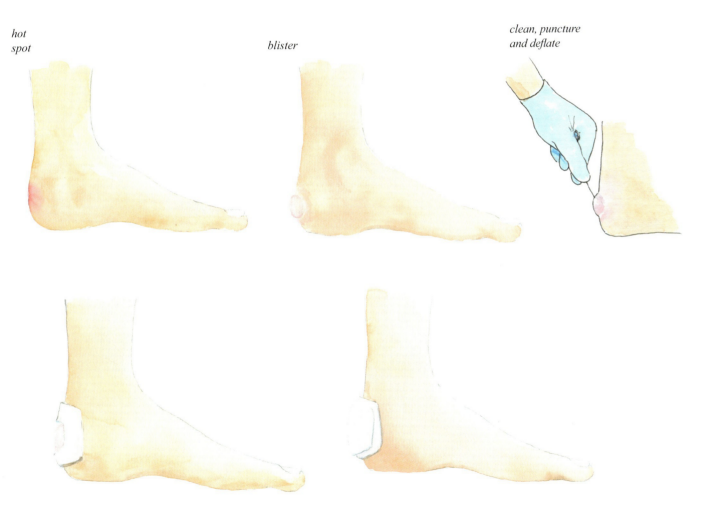

hot spot

blister

clean, puncture and deflate

protect with donut padding; fill donut hole with antibiotic ointment

protect and cover

SOFT TISSUE INJURIES:

BANDAGING SKILLS:

Dressing: Sterile material put directly onto a wound site.
- Sterile gauze pads: 2" x 2" or 4" x 4" trauma dressings.

Bandage: Piece of material that holds the dressings in place.
- Cravat: A large triangular piece of material that is used in very clever ways to hold dressings.
- ACE bandage: Elastic material 2" to 6" wide that can be used to hold dressings and also to apply compression.
- Roller gauze/ Kling: Soft, fluffy material in a roll, 1" to 6" wide that can be wrapped to hold a dressing in place.

Specific Bandages:

- **Scalp bandage**: To hold a dressing on the scalp.

- **Temporal/Jaw**: To hold a dressing on the side of the head, or to support the jaw.

- **Shoulder**: To hold a dressing on the shoulder or upper arm and maintain range of motion.

SOFT TISSUE INJURIES & MEDICAL EMERGENCIES

■ **Arm sling & swathe:** To support the shoulder, upper arm, elbow, forearm, or wrist.

■ **Hip**: To hold a dressing on the hip or buttocks and maintain full range of motion of the hip.

■ **Knee**: To hold a dressing on the knee and maintain full range of motion.

■ **Sprained ankle**: RICE
(If needed, use the ankle bandage shown in the Musculoskeletal chapter.)

81

MEDICAL EMERGENCIES & CRITICAL CARE:

These are rare but potentially life-threatening problems you need to be able to recognize and manage. A good history will usually make the diagnosis.

CHANGE IN LEVEL OF CONSCIOUSNESS:

Level of Consciousness (LOC) is maintained by the brain, so any change indicates a brain problem. Signs and Symptoms:

- ✓ Change in personality.
- ✓ Deteriorating LOC, A > V > P > U > **Death**
- ✓ Seizure activity.

Causes: Your brain needs four things to survive and thrive; causes of change in LOC:

- ✓ Oxygen (hypoxia).
- ✓ Carbohydrates (glucose, hypo/hyperglycemia).
- ✓ Proper temperature, $98.6°F/37°C$ (hypo/hyperthermia).
- ✓ Proper pressure = intracranial pressure (ICP).

Principles of Management

- ✓ Maintain and monitor the airway & breathing.
- ✓ Place in the Recovery Position to protect the airway.
- ✓ If respiratory rate less than 10 or greater than 30, assist breathing—1 breath every 5 seconds.
- ✓ Recognize the problem early and evacuate early as these problems tend to steadily deteriorate.
- ✓ If suspicious of a diabetic emergency, give them sugar.
- ✓ Get help; this patient needs to be evacuated ASAP.

SOFT TISSUE INJURIES & MEDICAL EMERGENCIES

SHORTNESS OF BREATH (SOB)—AIRWAY, BREATHING:

- The brain perceives that it is not getting enough oxygen so it causes a sensation of SOB.
- So, either there is not enough oxygen getting into the blood, or there is not enough oxygenated blood getting to the brain.

Signs and Symptoms:
- Complaining of shortness of breath.
- Rapid shallow or deep breathing.
- Skin color pale to cyanotic (blue) as hypoxia increases.
- May be wheezing.

Causes:
- Lungs: asthma (wheezing).
- Lungs: pneumothorax (no breath sounds on one side)
- Lungs: pulmonary edema, pneumonia (crackles).
- Lungs: pulmonary emboli (dyspnea).
- Heart: MI, angina (chest pain).
- Anaphylaxis, anxiety, altitude.

Principles of Management:

✓ **Look:** is your patient struggling to breathe—mouth open, obvious effort. Are they cyanotic; do they have hives?

✓ **Listen** to the breath sounds: is there wheezing, gurgling, or no breath sounds on one side?
- Support respirations; sitting up may help.
- Assist breathe for them if they cannot move enough air on their own.
- If asthmatic, may use **THEIR** rescue inhaler: Albuterol Metered Dose Inhaler (MDI), 2 puffs every 10 minutes until breathing improves (up to 4 times), then 2 puffs every 4 hours.

✓ If yes to these symptoms, get help—this patient needs to be evacuated **ASAP**.

ASTHMA

Allergens in the airway cause swelling, bronchospasm, and increased mucous production in the bronchioles. This causes the bronchioles to narrow resulting in wheezing, air trapping, and shortness of breath.

Signs and Symptoms:
- Shortness of breath.
- Word dyspnea—unable to count to ten on one breath.
- Expiratory wheezing—audible initially with auscultation.

Treatment:
- CALM the patient, and remain calm yourself.
- Place in position of comfort (usually sitting or semi-sitting).
- Take a good history—find out which medications, if any, have been taken.
- Assist with the use of rescue metered dose inhaler, Albuterol, or Xopenex.
- Encourage pursed-lip breathing to create backpressure and open bronchioles.
- May do lateral chest compressions to help remove trapped air.
- Consider evacuation.

CHEST PAIN:
- There are many harmless things that cause chest pain, such as indigestion, heartburn, pulled chest wall muscles.
- Your concern with chest pain is the chance that it is cardiac.

Signs and Symptoms (cardiac):
- Left-sided, substernal chest pain that may radiate into the left arm.
- Associated with a sensation of shortness of breath.
- Associated with a cold sweat.
- Is made worse by exertion and anxiety.

Causes:
- Non-cardiac: indigestion, heartburn, pulled muscles.
- Cardiac: acute MI, angina.

Principles of Management for Suspected Cardiac Pain:

✓ Goal is to minimize heart effort and strain.

✓ Unless you are absolutely certain that the pain is not cardiac, evacuate.

✓ The cardiac patient should be kept at rest, as exertion will make the pain worse.

✓ Transport in a position of comfort to support breathing.

SOFT TISSUE INJURIES & MEDICAL EMERGENCIES

✔ Keep them calm, reassure.

✔ If you have aspirin with you, give them 1 adult (325mg) or 4 baby aspirin (unless allergic to aspirin).

✔ Get help; this patient needs to be evacuated **ASAP**.

ANAPHYLACTIC REACTION:

- Is a severe, life-threatening allergic reaction.

Signs and Symptoms:
- The patient usually knows if they are allergic and will tell you (but ask anyway).
- They may have a rash—hives.
- They may have increasing shortness of breath.
- They may feel increasingly anxious, even terrified.
- They may wheeze and/or have difficulty breathing or speaking.

Causes:
- Bee stings (Hymenoptera: bees, wasps, hornets, fire ants).
- Foods, especially peanuts or seafood.
- Medications, e.g. penicillin.

Principles of Management:

✔ Immediately give antihistamine: Benadryl, 50mg every 4 hours for 24 hours; other antihistamines will also work.

✔ If they begin to lose their airway (SOB, wheezing), give epinephrine with an Epi-Pen or Twinject.

✔ Once able to breathe and swallow, give them the antihistamine as explained above.

✔ A second dose of epinephrine may be given if the first dose wears off before the antihistamine is absorbed.

✔ Evacuate immediately.

APPENDICES

SOLO—A LOOK AT WHO WE ARE

SOLO took root in the early 1970s and grew out of the vision of its founders, Frank Hubbell and Lee Frizzell (husband and wife). At that time, pre-hospital care was in its infancy, and an organized EMS system didn't exist yet in New Hampshire. The concept of providing emergency care to the sick and injured revolved around what is today referred to as the "Golden Hour." As injured skiers, climbers, and EMTs in the White Mountains of New Hampshire were being rescued, it very quickly became apparent that the skills that rescuers had learned as 'street emergency care providers did not work in a remote environment. It was obvious that people providing care in remote environments had to learn how to use skills and techniques outside the "golden hour." But, that information was not available—it had to be learned through experience. And Frank Hubbell had a great deal of experience, having been actively involved in Search and Rescue missions during college.

Frank's frustration with the lack of an appropriate "wilderness" standard led to the creation of one of the first, if not the first, organized wilderness/remote emergency medicine courses in the world. By 1975, a basic "Mountain/Woods First Aid" course was taken on the road by Frank, and that course outline and objectives remain the foundation of SOLO's most popular course today, Wilderness First Aid. The WFA class has been adapted for a number of specialized situations like water, disaster, and expedition.

SOLO's Main Building, Kaila Hall

In 1976, Frank, and his wife Lee Frizzell, a trained educator, created a school to develop and teach various aspects and levels of wilderness/remote/disaster medicine. They named that school SOLO, for Stonehearth Open Learning Opportunities.

At the beginning SOLO ran more than 30 courses for a variety of organizations, especially large outdoor organizations and colleges. Testimonials from these groups as to the importance and effectiveness of these programs provided proof that this type of training was essential, and SOLO began to create more programs tying them to national certifications whenever possible. Their courses became industry standards over the next decade. Word of these courses spread throughout the outdoor education industry, the environmental groups, and even the US Military and various government agencies. Students attending courses ranged in age from 16 to 70, coming from diverse backgrounds and careers, laypeople and medical professionals alike.

In 1982, Frank decided to further his medical education becoming a Physician Assistant, in 1984. During this time, SOLO founded the Wilderness Medicine Newsletter, and the staff not only published articles in that and other major EMS journals but presented at all major outdoor conferences.

SOLO founder Frank Hubbell teaching in 1980

• In 1988, SOLO staff helped develop wilderness clinical guidelines through the American Society for Testing and Materials (ASTM) Wilderness Medical Task Group. These guidelines were later adopted by the National Association of EMS Physicians. SOLO also participated in other consensus curriculum development groups with the growing number of programs, most of which, ironically had their roots in SOLO training

• At this same time, SOLO was featured in a Turner Broadcasting Systems programs as one of New Hampshire's as unique businesses.

• 1990 was another busy year, highlighted by publication of the first edition of the book "Medicine for the Backcountry" by Frank Hubbell and Buck Tilton and

• Through the next two decades SOLO received accreditation from several colleges so their graduates could receive college credit.

• Entering medical school in 1987, Frank graduated with several academic awards and "Graduate with Distinction honors.

- In 1998, SOLO was featured in the Encyclopedia Britannica's "Health and Medicine" supplement, and in 1999, we were the focus of a Time magazine column.
- 2001 marked SOLO's official 25th anniversary.
- Highlights of 2004, included SOLO's being featured in several PBS ventures (Through the years SOLO has been featured in several TV programs); SOLO's WEMT course receiving licensure from the State of New Hampshire's Postsecondary School Commission; Frank Hubbell being the recipient of NH's prestigious David J. Connor EMS Appreciation Award in recognition of his long-term dedication to NH's Emergency Medical Services; and SOLO's being honored with the "Educator of the Year" award at the Northern New Hampshire's EMS Conference.
- The release of a TMC illustrated book was a highpoint of 2005. The book was widely praised for its literary and artistic merit, was called one of the "Best Outdoor Books of 2005" by the chairman of the National Outdoor Book Awards, and went on to win five national book awards.
- The Wilderness Medicine Newsletter (WMN) continued to grow, both in size and distribution, as people responded to the new online format—which makes the WMN available anywhere in the world at the click of a mouse.
- The 2005 January issue of Outside Magazine mentioned SOLO courses in an article entitled "50 Ways to Live Large" as one of the 50 experiences from around the world that you need to participate in before you die, and AMC Outdoors featured a piece on the SOLO Wilderness First Responder program in their November 2005 issue.

 By the end of the year. TMC had published the full set of NH State EMS Protocols at the request of the state of NH and has continued to update these for NH every other year since.

- From 2006 into the present, SOLO has enlarged its out-of-country trainings, providing courses in Tanzania, Kenya, Zambia, Turkey, Israel, Chile, Mexico, Costa Rica, Indonesia, Scotland, Haiti… More partnerships are being formed as programs for indigenous people have become an important focus for SOLO. Following the earthquake in Haiti, teams from SOLO made trips to that devastated nation for several months to assist in urban clinics, hospitals and rural medical centers. A specialized set of programs under the umbrella of GeoMed has been developed to better serve the needs of people in more remote areas or disaster situations.

Thirty-eight years after the official founding of SOLO, interest in wilderness/remote/disaster medicine training is still growing. Nine month-long WEMT courses are offered on our campus annually along with several dozen other programs.

Hundreds of other programs continue to be offered worldwide with much of the emphasis now on the disaster side of long-term care. Since SOLO has been a licensed NH rescue unit for years, our staff and students volunteer on backcountry search and rescue missions in NH's White Mountains.

From a gathering in a living room over almost four decades, SOLO has grown into a large, diverse organization: a leader not only in medicine, but also in education and standards as well. From basic first aid—still the foundation of SOLO's purpose—we now find instructors teaching around the country as well as internationally, reaching outdoor users, trip leaders, expeditioners, and people far from help. By the end of 2014, well over 310,000 people will have taken a SOLO class.

APPENDICES

Part I quiz: Response and Assessment   **Student Name** _____

1. Which of the following are common modes of transmission of infectious disease?
   - ☐ a. Airborne by inhaling infectious particles.
   - ☐ b. Vector or insect bite.
   - ☐ c. Waterborne by drinking contaminated water.
   - ☐ d. Direct contact or bloodborne.
   - ☐ e. All of the above.

2. The purpose of the Primary Survey is all of the following except:
   - ☐ a. Find and treat all potentially life-threatening problems.
   - ☐ b. Protect from the environment.
   - ☐ c. Prevent any further injury.
   - ☐ d. Establish and monitor vital signs.

3. The Secondary Survey consists of:
   - ☐ a. Vital signs.
   - ☐ b. Patient exam.
   - ☐ c. AMPLE history.
   - ☐ d. SOAPNOTE.
   - ☐ e. All of the above.

4. All of the following AMPLE history explanations are correct except for:
   - ☐ a. A = allergies.
   - ☐ b. M = medications.
   - ☐ c. P = previous injuries or illness.
   - ☐ d. L = last in and out.
   - ☐ e. E = environmental conditions.

5. The Objective part of the SOAPnote will contain all of the following except:
   - ☐ a. Heart rate, respiratory rate and effort, & level of consciousness.
   - ☐ b. Description of locations of pain, tenderness, and injuries.
   - ☐ c. AMPLE history.
   - ☐ d. Condition of the group as a whole.

6. The rescue plan consists of all of the following except:
   - ☐ a. The group's condition.
   - ☐ b. Treating the patient's injuries.
   - ☐ c. The group's level of preparedness.
   - ☐ d. Sending for help.

Part II quiz: Trauma: Musculoskeletal Injuries:

Student Name _____

1. A sprain or strain can cause injury to all of the following except:
   - ☐ a. Muscle.
   - ☐ b. Tendon.
   - ☐ c. Ligament.
   - ☐ d. Bone.

2. All of the following are correct for treating a sprain except:
   - ☐ a. Rest, stop, and sit down.
   - ☐ b. Ice for vasoconstriction.
   - ☐ c. Compression with an ACE bandage.
   - ☐ d. Elevation to decrease circulation to the affected area.
   - ☐ e. Mild exercise to encourage healing.

3. Which of the following statements regarding fractures is correct?
   - ☐ a. There is typically point tenderness over the fracture site.
   - ☐ b. The patient may have felt something snap, crack, or pop.
   - ☐ c. There may be discoloration, swelling, or deformity.
   - ☐ d. There is a loss of normal function.
   - ☐ e. All are correct.

4. The most important aspect of fracture care is to:
   - ☐ a. Maintain normal function and range of motion.
   - ☐ b. Maintain circulation distal to the site of the injury.
   - ☐ c. Adjust the fracture site until there is normal sensation and movement.
   - ☐ d. Splint the fracture exactly the way you found it.

5. The reason to straighten out an angulated fracture is to:
   - ☐ a. Make it easier to splint.
   - ☐ b. Place the injury in a more comfortable position.
   - ☐ c. Establish and maintain circulation.
   - ☐ d. Place it in the proper position for healing.

6. Splints should be monitored every 15 minutes to:
   - ☐ a. Make sure that the splint is still tight and snug.
   - ☐ b. Make sure the fracture is in the proper position.
   - ☐ c. Make sure the extremity is staying cool so that it will not swell.
   - ☐ d. Make sure there is circulation distal to the fracture.

7. Which of the following statements is incorrect regarding spinal injuries?
   - ☐ a. The patient must by sober and oriented x 3 to "clear" the spine.
   - ☐ b. The patient should be free of distracting injuries at the time of the exam.
   - ☐ c. If they fell more than twice their height, you must treat for a back injury.
   - ☐ d. You can move the patient from position of injury to position of function.

Part III quiz: Environmental Emergencies   Student Name _____

Circle True or False in regard to the following statements about hypothermia:
- T / F   Hypothermia is most commonly associated with cold, wet, windy conditions.
- T / F   Humans are designed to lose heat when wet.
- T / F   Hypothermia has little or no effect on the human brain.
- T / F   Humans burn glucose as a fuel to help maintain body temperature.
- T / F   Shivering is involuntary muscular contractions that produce heat.
- T / F   Shivering does NOT impair other physical activity.
- T / F   Conscious hypothermia victims need water and glucose.
- T / F   Never expose and dry off a wet hypothermia patient.

Which of the following is incorrect regarding frostbite?
- ☐ a. Superficial frostbite can be field rewarmed with skin-to-skin contact.
- ☐ b. Deep frostbite should not be field rewarmed, but should be protected from further damage.
- ☐ c. Refreezing recently thawed frostbite will cause a much worse injury.
- ☐ d. It is preferable to use hot air to thaw frostbitten hands.

Which of the following is correct regarding heat stroke?
- ☐ a. Heat stroke is a minor injury associated with dehydration and salt depletion.
- ☐ b. Heat stroke is self-correcting and does not require treatment.
- ☐ c. Heat stroke patients need to be aggressively cooled with water.
- ☐ d. Heat stroke is rarely associated with dehydration.

When someone is sent out to get help, all of the following are true except:
- ☐ a. Keep everyone busy, and keep everyone warm and dry.
- ☐ b. Build a bivouac to protect the patient and everyone else in the group.
- ☐ c. Build a fire or light a stove to make something warm to drink.
- ☐ d. Send someone out for help every 1 – 2 hours until help arrives.

Part IV quiz: Soft Tissue Injuries and Critical Care   Student Name _____

1. All of the following statements are correct except:
   - ☐ a. Blood is sterile and harmless to others exposed to it.
   - ☐ b. Arteries are under pressure, and although rare, spurt blood when cut.
   - ☐ c. Veins are low pressure and drain blood when cut.
   - ☐ d. Capillaries are very small and low pressure; they ooze or seep when cut.
   - ☐ e. Veins are commonly injured because they can be just under the skin.

2. All of the following statements about controlling bleeding are correct except:
   - ☐ a. Pressure directly over the wound is the most effective way to control bleeding.
   - ☐ b. If direct pressure is not enough, you can also elevate the wound.
   - ☐ c. Pressure dressings are very effective but should only be used for about 10 minutes.
   - ☐ d. Never remove a dressing once it has been placed on the wound.
   - ☐ e. In extreme cases direct digital pressure can be applied directly to an open spurting artery.

3. All of the following are signs or symptoms of a localized tissue infection except:
   - ☐ a. The area is red (rubor).
   - ☐ b. The area is warm to the touch (calor).
   - ☐ c. The area is swollen (tumor).
   - ☐ d. The area is tender to the touch (dolor).
   - ☐ e. The area is red but not warm to the touch.

4. Please answer True or False about severe potentially life-threatening tissue infections:
   - T / F   There can be a collection of pus or other drainage coming from the wound.
   - T / F   There may be red streaks running proximally from the infection site.
   - T / F   There may be swollen tender lymph nodes proximal to the infection site.
   - T / F   The patient may have fever and chills.
   - T / F   Wound infections can be prevented by proper cleaning and bandaging.
   - T / F   Wounds associated with impairment of circulation, sensation, or movement do not need to be immediately evacuated; they can wait 2 – 3 days.

5. Which statement is incorrect in regard to impaled objects?
   - ☐ a. Never remove impaled objects.
   - ☐ b. Remove impaled objects that are in an extremity.
   - ☐ c. Remove metal impaled objects in a cold environment.
   - ☐ d. Do not remove impaled objects in the skull, neck, chest, or abdomen.

6. Which of the following statements is incorrect about thermal burns.
   - ☐ a. Immediately cold soak the burn area with cold water for about 15 minutes.
   - ☐ b. Superficial burns rarely cause very much pain.
   - ☐ c. Deep burns have minimal pain due to nerve destruction in the skin.
   - ☐ d. All deep burns patients need to be hydrated and evacuated.

SOAPNOTE

Subjective: age, sex, mechanism of injury (MOI), chief complaint(C/C): _____
_____
_____
_____
_____

Objective: vital signs, patient exam, AMPLE history:

Vital Signs

TIME					
LOC oriented x ?					
RR & effort					
HR & effort					
Skin C, T, M					

Patient Exam: Describe locations of pain, tenderness & injuries:

Allergies:
Medications: _____
Past pertinent medical history: _____
Last in and out: _____
Events leading up to accident:
_____

Assessment: problem list:
1. _____
2. _____
3. _____

Plan: plan for each problem on the problem list:
1. _____
2. _____
3. _____
4. MONITOR - How often do you plan to monitor the patient? _____

© 2007 SOLO

SOAPNOTE

Subjective: age, sex, mechanism of injury (MOI), chief complaint(C/C): _____
_____
_____
_____

Objective: vital signs, patient exam, AMPLE history:

Vital Signs

TIME					
LOC oriented x ?					
RR & effort					
HR & effort					
Skin C, T, M					

Patient Exam: Describe locations of pain, tenderness & injuries:

Allergies:
Medications:_____
Past pertinent medical history:_____
Last in and out:_____
Events leading up to accident:
_____

Assessment: problem list:
1._____
2._____
3._____

Plan: plan for each problem on the problem list:
1._____
2._____
3._____
4. MONITOR - How often do you plan to monitor the patient? _____

© 2007 SOLO

APPENDICES

SOAPNOTE

Subjective: age, sex, mechanism of injury (MOI), chief complaint(C/C): _____
_____
_____
_____
_____

Objective: vital signs, patient exam, AMPLE history:

Vital Signs

TIME					
LOC oriented x ?					
RR & effort					
HR & effort					
Skin C, T, M					

Patient Exam: Describe locations of pain, tenderness & injuries:

Allergies:
Medications: _____
Past pertinent medical history: _____
Last in and out: _____
Events leading up to accident:

Assessment: problem list:
1. _____
2. _____
3. _____

Plan: plan for each problem on the problem list:
1. _____
2. _____
3. _____
4. MONITOR - How often do you plan to monitor the patient? _____

© 2007 SOLO

SOAPNOTE

Subjective: age, sex, mechanism of injury (MOI), chief complaint(C/C): _____
_____
_____
_____

Objective: vital signs, patient exam, AMPLE history:

Vital Signs

TIME					
LOC oriented x ?					
RR & effort					
HR & effort					
Skin C, T, M					

Patient Exam: Describe locations of pain, tenderness & injuries:

Allergies:
Medications:_____
Past pertinent medical history:_____
Last in and out:_____
Events leading up to accident:
_____

Assessment: problem list:
1._____
2._____
3._____

Plan: plan for each problem on the problem list:
1._____
2._____
3._____
4. MONITOR - How often do you plan to monitor the patient? _____

© 2007 SOLO

Upon successful completion of this course you will be able to perform:

Patient Assessment System and Critical Care

    Scene Survey – Scene Safety

    Primary Survey – Life Threats

    Secondary Survey

    Rescue Survey

    Shock – recognition and treatment of shock

Trauma: Musculoskeletal Injuries – Recognition and Treatment of:

    Sprain and strains and Fractures

    Upper extremity injuries:

        Sling and Swathe

        Forearm/wrist splint

    Lower leg and knee injuries:

        Lower leg and knee splints

Soft Tissue and Medical Emergencies:

    Control of Bleeding

    Long-term wound care

    Bandaging skills:

        Scalp bandage

        Temporal bandage

        Arm sling and swathe

        Shoulder and hip bandage

        Knee bandage

        Sprained ankle bandage

    Thermal burn care

    Blister care

Medical Emergencies – Recognition and Management of:

    Change in Level Of Consciousness

    Chest pain

    Shortness of breath and Asthma

    Anaphylaxis

Environmental Emergencies – Recognition and Management of:

    Hypothermia and Frostbite

    Heat Stroke, Heat Exhaustion, and dehydration

    North American Bites and Stings

    Lightning

    Bivouac and Survival Skills

SOLO

We hope that you enjoy our SOLO course. SOLO is the nation's leader in wilderness medicine education with over 300,000 students attending courses since 1976. SOLO has been instrumental in the development of Wilderness First Aid, Wilderness First Responder, and Wilderness EMT curricula. Our campus, perched on 300 acres in the heart of New Hampshire's White Mountains, is a unique teaching facility made up of our three-story Main Building, a 30-person dorm, dining hall, and other facilities. Find out more about SOLO by visiting soloschools.com. We hope you decide to continue your wilderness medicine education by attending one of our other programs. SOLO, PO Box 3150, Conway, NH 03818 • 603-447-6711

WMN *Wilderness Medicine Newsletter*

The Wilderness Medicine Newsletter

Always late, always worth the wait!

Subscriptions $15 a year.
www.wildernessmedicinenewsletter.com

SOLO has produced the *Wilderness Medicine Newsletter* continuously since 1988. It is dedicated to disseminating information on medical issues and practices in the backcountry. The newsletter is a full-color online journal. Subscribers have access to all back issues to 2002. Learn all about the newsletter and get more information by visiting us at tmcbooks.com.

For more information on any of our programs just go to our website:

www.soloschools.com

Now that you have just completed your Wilderness First Aid course, you are probably excited to learn more. GREAT!

We wanted to reward you for a job well done by offering you a discount for the Wilderness First Responder (WFR) course or the Wilderness EMT (WEMT) course on the SOLO campus in Conway, New Hampshire.

This gift certificate is only for SOLO WFA graduates. It is are non-transferable. You may apply this $50 (fifty) coupon towards the WFR course, or you may apply this as a $100 (one hundred) coupon towards the WEMT course.

When you sign up for a WFR or WEMT course and want to apply the coupon, please give the registrar your name, the date when you took the WFA course, and where you took the WFA course. You will need to send a copy of your WFA certification in with your course registration. Please contact us if you have any questions at (603) 447-6711

Thanks again for joining us for a SOLO WFA course!